THE ULTIMATE LOW-FODMAP DIET COOKBOOK

1000 Days Complete Simple & Delicious Recipes to Manage Digestive Disorders and Relieve IBS – 30-Day meal plan

TYLER RUIZ

TABLE OF CONTENTS

INTRODUCTION

The Ultimate Low-FODMAP Diet Cookbook is a comprehensive guide to managing digestive disorders such as the symptoms of irritable bowel syndrome (IBS) with a particular diet. The Low-FODMAP eating plan is a proven method for reducing symptoms such as bloating, gas, and abdominal pain by limiting the consumption of certain carbohydrates that can be difficult to digest.

This cookbook is designed to make it easy for anyone following the Low-FODMAP diet to enjoy delicious and varied meals every day of the year. With 365 recipes, there is something for everyone, from hearty breakfasts and tasty snacks to satisfying dinners and indulgent desserts. Each recipe in this cookbook is carefully crafted to be Low-FODMAP compliant while still being flavorful and satisfying. The recipes are straightforward to follow and have clear instructions and ingredient lists. In addition, the cookbook includes tips and tricks for meal planning and preparation, making it a valuable resource for anyone seeking to manage their digestive disorder through diet.

Whether you are new to the Low-FODMAP diet or have been following it for some time, The Ultimate Low-FODMAP Diet Cookbook is an essential addition to your kitchen. With this cookbook, you can enjoy delicious meals daily while managing your digestive disorder and improving your overall health and well-being.

CHAPTER 1

FODMAP

FODMAP diet approach is Fermentable Oligosaccharides, Disaccharides, and Polyols, is an abbreviations for these substances. These carbs may be found in a wide variety of meals, including grains, dairy items, fruits, vegetables, and sweets.

These carbohydrates may not be well absorbed in certain individuals' small intestines, passing instead into the

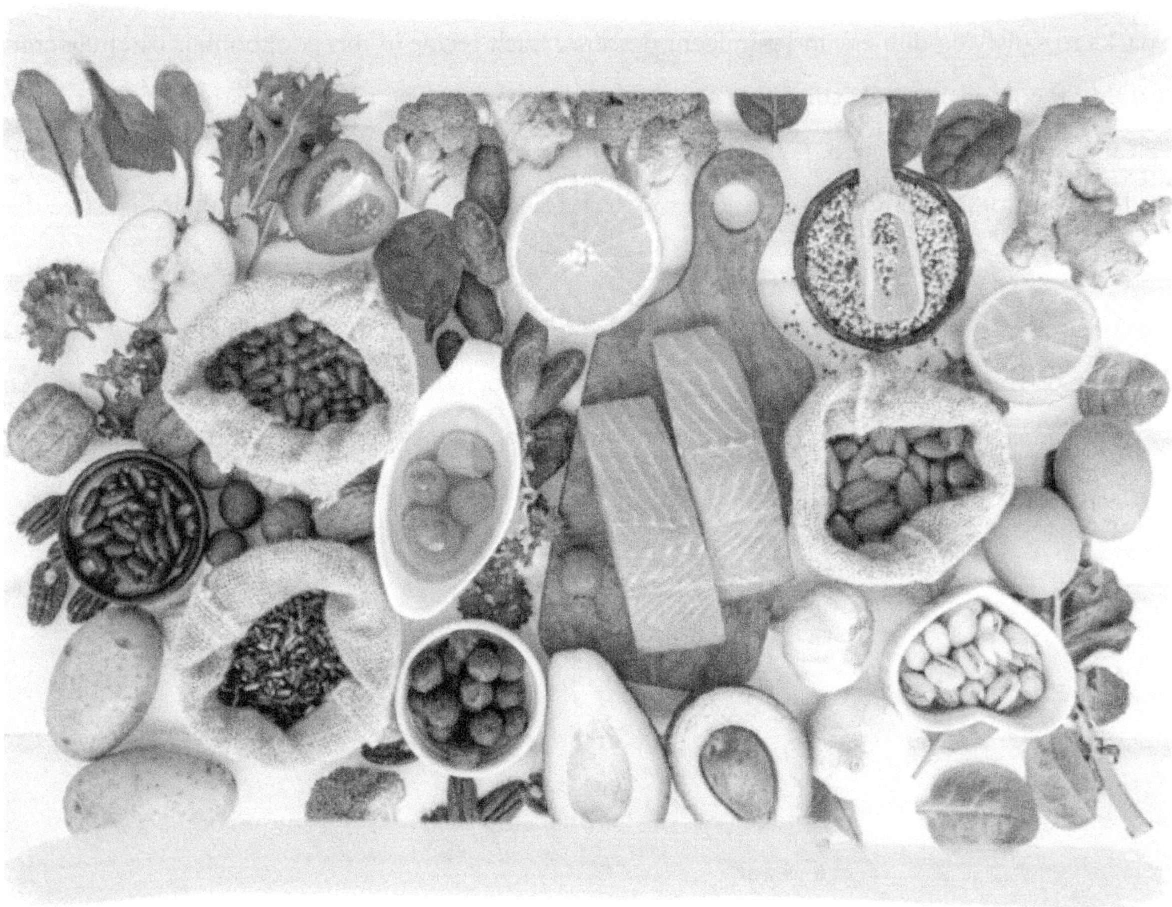

large intestine, where they are digested by bacteria. Gas production, bloating, pain in the abdomen, diarrhea, or constipation may result from this fermentation.

The Low-FODMAP diet is a dietary strategy created to treat the signs and symptoms of digestive problems such inflammatory bowel disease. illness and irritable bowel syndrome (IBD, IBS). The diet involves reducing or eliminating high-FODMAP foods from the diet for some time and then gradually reintroducing them to identify specific trigger foods. Low-FODMAP foods, such as rice, oats, quinoa, potatoes, carrots, green beans, bananas, strawberries, and lactose-free dairy, can be consumed without symptoms.

The Low-FODMAP diet aims to help people with digestive disorders identify and manage foods that trigger symptoms while maintaining adequate nutrient intake. However, working with a healthcare provider or registered dietitian is essential to ensure the diet is properly balanced and sustainable for the individual's needs.

Should you try a Low FODMAP diet?

Because so many people have sensitivities to the foods that fall into the categories mentioned above, an effective IBS diet plan that may significantly improve your general quality of life and, consequently, the health of your digestive system can be created with the use of an elimination diet. But, like any elimination diet, it can significantly change your general well-being; hence the low FODMAP diet is only suitable for some.

The low FODMAP diet might not be the most effective treatment for individuals with Celiac disease, even though they're beneficial for those with gluten sensitivity since they seek to eliminate glucose, not gluten. Therefore they may still include trigger foods. Yet, they can be effective for those sensitive to, even though they do not have celiac disease, gluten, as the FODMAPs in wheat may trigger this delicacy. Also, it is not the best course of action for underweight individuals or having eating problems.

Suppose you have preexisting health issues or think you could be suffering from an unidentified digestive disorder. In such a situation, see your doctor before beginning any elimination diet, such as the low FODMAP diet. It is a good idea.

CHAPTER 2

LOW-FODMAP DIET

A FODMAP-restricted Elimination dieting is a type of diet. Some such elimination diets are the allergy diet, the ketogenic diet, the paleo diet, and the autoimmune paleo diet (AIP). All elimination diets start with the premise that particular foods or dietary groups are to blame for specific adverse reactions and symptoms. Many elimination diets aim to reduce autoimmune indicators and flare-ups, so you may reintroduce or increase

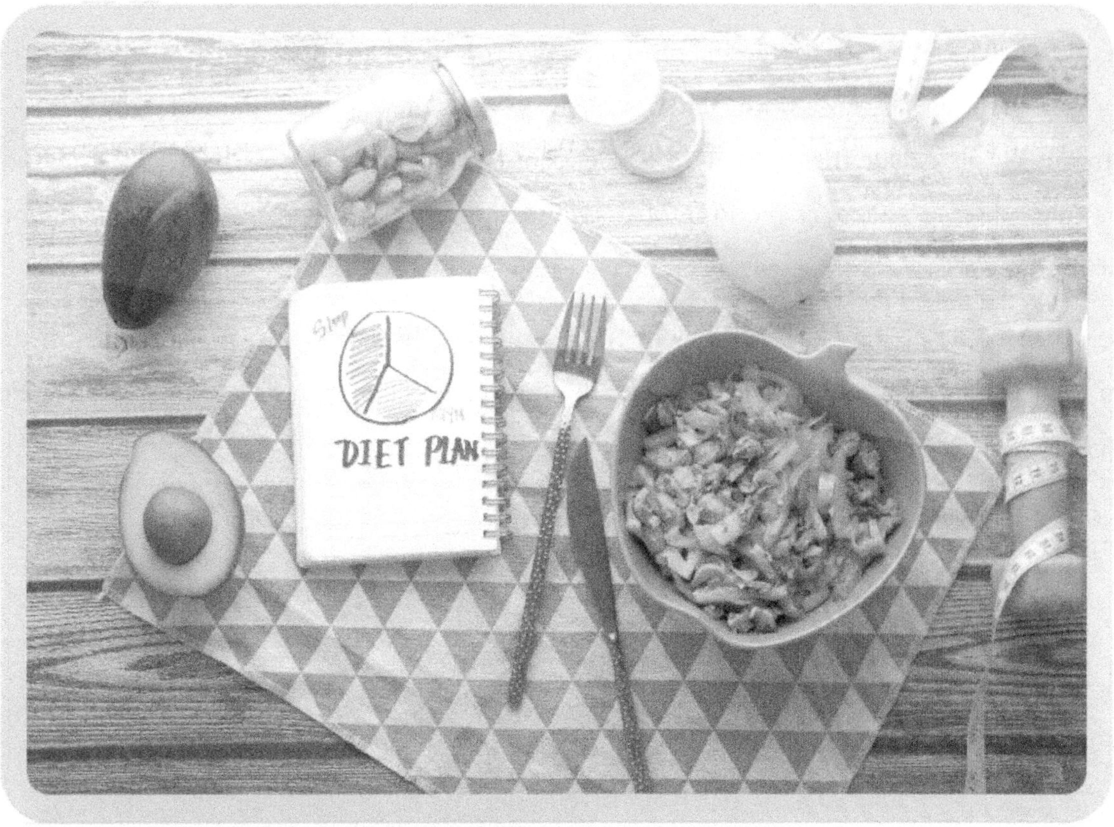

your intake of these items to see which ones have an adverse effect.

A low FODMAP diet is commonly utilized as part of the recovery plan for treating SIBO (small intestinal bacterial overgrowth) or IBS (irritable bowel syndrome) (SIBO).

The low FODMAP diet is a three-pronged strategy for treating digestive disorders: restriction, elimination, and gradual reintroduction.

To what do the letters FODMAP refer?

The abbreviation for "fermentable oligo-, di-, mono-, and polyols" is "FODMAP." In other words, sugars and starches:

- Fruits, sweet meals, and even certain vegetables contain fructose.
- Dairy products include lactose.
- Grains are an excellent source of fructans.
- Beans and lentils are good sources of galanin.
- Xylitol, sorbitol, and maltitol are all examples of sugar alcohols that contain polyols.

Problems with digestion may result from the increased resistance to digestion posed by these short-chain carbohydrates. They move gradually through the intestine, causing a buildup of fluid. They ferment when entering the digestive tract, leading to unpleasant symptoms like abdominal pain, gas, bloating, and even diarrhea. Many people can tolerate FODMAPS just fine, even if they have these symptoms. Those with SIBO and IBS may want to try a low FODMAP diet to determine if these items cause discomfort.

The FODMAP Scale

High-FODMAP foods are those that are high in these particular carbs. Each food is assigned a score based on how high in FODMAPs it is. The red, orange, or green classification of a food can help determine how frequently it should be consumed, which foods should be avoided, and which meals should be considered important staples. The quantity consumed or the cooking process might affect a food's quality.

In which cases could a low-FODMAP diet be helpful?

Those people most likely to gain from a low FODMAP diet are those with irritable bowel syndrome (IBS) or small intestinal bacterial overgrowth (SIBO). Individuals that struggle with gastrointestinal issues like bloating, gas, indigestion, and diarrhea may find relief on a low FODMAP diet.

- Garlic and onions are high in fermentable oligosaccharides and polyols (FOD).
- Beans, lentils, and other pulses
- Bread and muffins made with wheat flour or rye (in considerable quantities)
- Fruits & Veggies: Watermelon, peaches, apples, cherries, nectarines, pears, mango, avocados, sugar snap peas, green peas, artichokes, and asparagus.
- Sausage, breaded fish/ meat, and steak are examples of meat and protein.
- Almonds, cashews, and pistachios

- Plain cow's milk-based yogurt, ice cream, and custard;
- Honey and high fructose corn syrup combined;

Including Protein Into Low FODMAP

- Diets: We eat a wide variety of foods, including (fermented soy)
- The vast majority of edible fats and oils, peanuts
- Vegetables and Fruits: bananas, melons (apart from watermelon), (except kiwi, grapes, citrus, onions, artichokes, and other members of the cruciferous family (lime, lemon, grapefruit, etc.)
- Grains: rice, quinoa, corn, oats, and
- Dairy products: Lactose-free milk, ice cream, yogurt, and cheeses including Brie, Camembert, and Feta.
- Sugar, rice malt syrup, maple syrup, and dark chocolate
- Bread with a moderate amount of sourdough starter
- Beverages: Caffeine and Herbal Tea

For the most part, a low FODMAP diet consists of the intake of nuts, seeds, fruits, and lipids, with the exception of those you should stay away from, such as watermelon, cashews, and pistachios. These amazing foods are often great prebiotics for those without irritable bowel syndrome. Otherwise, they are known to be beneficial for intestinal health. If in doubt, you should always double-check, but soon you will be an expert!

Items to avoid while following a low-FODMAP diet.

There are several common high FODMAP foods that many people with IBS might be triggered by, even if the precise kind and quantity of FODMAPs your tailored elimination plan avoids may vary from others. They consist of:

- Milk, Yoghurt, Soy milk;
- Wheat, rye, beans, and chickpeas;
- Fruits including watermelon, avocados, and cherries;
- Vegetables including cabbage, beets, broccoli, and asparagus
- High-fructose corn syrup-containing soft drinks
- Apple juice
- Espresso coffee from machine

- Agave
- Xylitol

Instructions for Beginning and Maintaining diet low in FODMAPs

As been previously stated, low FODMAP diet plan may be broken down into three simple phases. The Monash FODMAP Diet provides more information at the link below.

Step one: Discard

It is recommended to start the low-FODMAP diet for two to six weeks. While the method is straightforward, it does call for some study. To start, try switching to low-FODMAP foods instead of their high-FODMAP counterparts. The recommended course of action is to consume foods with a low FODMAP ranking and avoid those with a moderate FODMAP rating.

The Monash traffic light system will aid in your education. What foods have the highest or lowest FODMAP content? This tool is great for reintroduction, personalization, and a new diet.

The ideal result throughout this period is for IBS symptoms to improve or go away. If so, you may move on to the following stage, allowing you to better grasp problematic foods. It's possible that FODMAPs aren't making your symptoms worse. You should think about other therapy options in this case.

Second step: Reintroduction

The period of reintroduction comes next. The objective is to get knowledge of specific FODMAP triggers. One carbohydrate type will be reintroduced at a time. To figure this out. You must pick meals that contain only one FODMAP and none of the others, so here is where a good guide will come in handy. This meal will treat symptoms for up to three days to see if they trigger an IBS flare-up or aggravate existing ones.

You can use the FODMAP challenges in the Monash FODMAP app to get help with step two. Also, it has a feature for keeping track of symptoms in a journal.

Step Three – Personalization

Here, you make semi-permanent modifications. The goal of any elimination diet is to keep eating as many foods as possible that don't have any negative side effects so you may have the greatest life possible while cooking and eating! You'll discover which meals may be enjoyed as treats and which cannot. Poorly tolerated foods should be avoided or reserved for use in upcoming FODMAP challenges to track any potential changes, while well-tolerated meals should take precedence.

Benefits of a low-FODMAP diet for health

Diet low in FODMAP is a therapeutic diet that involves limiting or avoiding foods high in fermentable carbohydrates that can cause digestive symptoms such as bloating, gas, and abdominal pain. In addition to polyols, fermentable oligosaccharides, disaccharides, monosaccharides, and class of carbohydrates (FODMAPs) might be problematic for some people's digestive systems.

The benefits of the Low-FODMAP diet include:

It reduces symptoms of intestinal illnesses such Crohn's disease, ulcerative colitis, and irritable bowel syndrome (IBS).

It identifies specific trigger foods that cause symptoms.

We are improving the overall quality of life by reducing digestive symptoms and improving bowel habits.

CHAPTER 3

BREAKFAST RECIPES

3.1 Granny Smith Apples

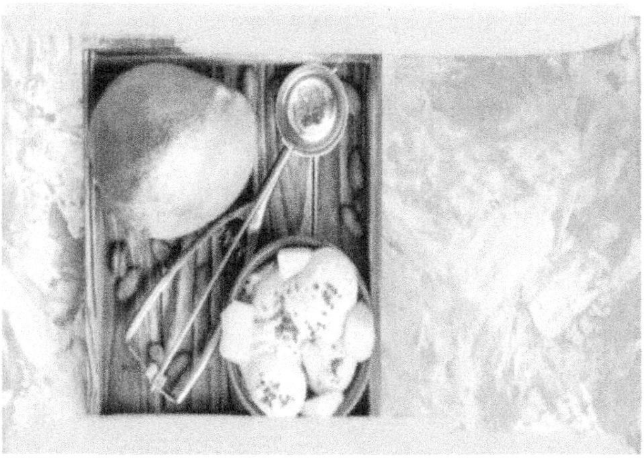

Time spent on preparation: 0 minutes

Time spent on cooking: 5 minutes

Degree of Difficulty: Simple

Serving: 2

Ingredients:

- 3/4 cup plain coffee almond milk
- A half cup raisin; 1 cup rolled oats;
- One quarter teaspoon cinnamon powder
- Two tablespoons of date · molasses or brown rice
- syrup

Directions:

In a large mixing basin, combine solid and liquid ingredients, and if you use date molasses. Stir to combine.

Grate the apple into the cereal when it's Time for

serve it, or slice and core it separately and then add it to the grain after giving it a good toss.

Nutritional Information: 118 calories, 13 g fat, 12 g amino, 7 g protein

---

3.2 Spiced Congee with Dates

Time spent on preparation: 0 minutes

Time spent on cooking: 5 minutes

Degree of Difficulty: Simple

Serving: 2

Ingredients:

- 4 cups brown rice, cooked
- Half cup (of each) date and apricot
- One cinnamon stick, big
- 1/4 teaspoon cloves, ground
- Season with salt to taste

Directions:

Over high heat, bring two and a half cups to a boil, bringing moderate water heat. Include fruits, cinnamon, rice, clove. Cook on a slow fire for fifteen mins.

Season with salt and pepper.

Nutritional Information: 148 calories, 13 g fat, 16 g amino, 22 g protein

---

3.3 Ham and Cheddar Omelets

Time spent on preparation: two minutes

Time spent on cooking: 20 minutes

Degree of difficulty: Easy

Serving: 2

Ingredients:

- Two steaks of ham
- One tablespoon of butter
- 1/2 onion (diced)
- One minced garlic clove
- Seven quail eggs
- One cup cheese, cheddar-type
- Half cup Heavy cooker's Cream
- To season, use Salt and pepper
- One tablespoon of chopped chives

Directions:

Set the oven's temperature to 400

Cube the fried ham steak.

Combine the eggs, salt, cream, and pepper. Compound should be smooth after being combined.

Add the ham in diced form.

In an oven-safe pan, melt the butter. After 2 minutes of onion and garlic frying, add the egg and the ham combination.

Bake for twenty minutes, or till golden brown, in the oven.

Add a final garnish of minced chives.

Nutritional Information: 302 calories, 13 g fat, 14 g amino, 20 g protein

---

3.4 Basic Oatmeal

Time spent on preparation: 0 mins

Time spent on cooking: 10 mins

Degree of difficulty: Easy

Serving: 2

Ingredients:

- 1 cup oats, rolled
- 2 cups water or vegetable milk
- Season with salt

Directions:

First, place a small saucepan on the stove and add

the vegetable milk, salt, and oatmeal. Once these ingredients are combined, bring the mixture to a boil.

Next, let it simmer gently and cook for about 5 minutes, till it becomes creamy.

Nutritional Information: 189 calories, 9 g fat, 12 g amino, 24 g protein

3.5 Chorizo, Tomato & Grill Chili Frittata

Time spent on preparation: 0 minutes

Time spent on cooking:.15 minutes

Degree of Difficulty: Easy to Moderate

Serving: 2

Ingredients:

- 6 oz. chorizo de Carne
- Eight oz. green chilli pepper (canned)
- 2/3 cup chopped/sliced red tomatoes
- Cheddar cheese, 2 oz.
- Eggs 3

Directions:

In a big nonstick pan, brown the beef and pork chorizo for approximately 5 minutes over moderate-high heat, breaking it up into bite-size pieces.

Remove and discard any surplus fat.

Prepare the broiler in the meanwhile.

Toss the chorizo in the pan with tomatoes, softly beaten eggs, cheese, and green chilies. Five minutes of high-heat cooking follows. Finish under the broiler for another 5 minutes or until slightly puffed.

Serve right away.

Nutritional Information: 203 calories, 10 g fat, 16 g amino, 24 g protein

---

3.6 Muesli with Coconut, Oats & Bananas

Time spent on preparation: 10 mins

Time spent on cooking: 10 mins

Degree of Difficulty: Easy

Serving: 2

Ingredients:

- 1 cup oats, rolled
- 3/4 cup almond milk, unsweetened
- Only half-cup dates
- A quarter cup of toasted unsweetened coconut
- one banana

Directions:

Combine and whisk all the fruits together and oats.

The last two minutes add the milk and whisk again, then add soak for 15 minutes.

Nutritional Information: 228 calories, 12 g fat, 12 g amino, 12 g protein

---

3.7 Steel-Cut Oats

Time spent on preparation: 0 mins

Time spent on cooking: 15 mins

Degree of Difficulty: Easy

Serving: 2

Ingredients:

- 1 cup oats, steel-cut
- 2 cups dried apple, chopped
- 1 cup pitted and chopped dates
- One stick of cinnamon

Directions:

Whisk cinnamon, oats, dates, apple, and 4 cups water in a slow-cooker.

Cook for at least 8 hours or until the oats are soft. Before serving, take off the cinnamon stick.

Nutritional Information: 202 calories, 13 g fat, 12 g amino, 24 g protein

---

3.8 Crumbles with Berries, Walnuts & Oats

Time spent on preparation: 0 mins

Time spent on cooking: 25 mins

Degree of Difficulty: Easy

Serving: 2

Ingredients:

- 1 & 1/2 tbsp. lemon juice
- One tea pour vanilla extract
- Cornstarch (two table pours)
- 4 cups thawed mixed berries, either fresh or frozen
- 2/3 cup oats (quick-cooking)
- 2 oz. walnuts, chopped
- 1 pound of stevia
- 1 tbsp. oil (canola)
- 1/2 tea pour the cinnamon powder
- A quarter tea pour of salt
- 1 cup plain Greek yoghurt

Directions:

Set the oven's temperature to 340 degrees Fahrenheit. In the meantime, mix the cornstarch, vanilla, along with lemon juice in a 2-quart casserole dish until the cornstarch is well incorporated. Mix thoroughly after adding the berries.

Combine the topping ingredients in a moderate mixing basin until crumbly.

Sprinkle evenly over the berries and bake for 30 minutes, uncovered.

Nutritional Information: 310 calories, 13 g fat, 13 g amino, 18 g protein

---

3.9 Breakfast Pancakes

Time spent on preparation: 10 mins

Time spent on cooking: 10 mins

Serving: 2

Degree of Difficulty: Easy

Ingredients:

- Bacon (four slices)
- 2 beaten egg whites
- 1/3 cup flour made from coconut
- One tablespoon of pure granular gelatin
- Two tablespoons unsalted butter, melted
- One tablespoon of finely chopped chives
- Filtered water, 1/3 cup

Directions:

Lay a pan on the stove and throw in the bacon, which you will cook with the fat that melts from it.

When it is slightly crispy, you can transfer it to a plate, having first covered it with a sheet of paper towels. Remember to leave the bacon fat in the pan because you will need it later.

Take the eggs, separate the yolk and white, and start beating only the whites with a hand blender.

Combine chives, gelatin, butter, coconut flour, and bacon in a mixing dish.

Pour the filtered water into the remaining ingredients and thoroughly mix it in.

Gently fold or whisk in the egg whites until well-integrated.

Melt the bacon grease in a pan.

Pour two tablespoons of the batter or mixture into the hot grease, smoothing it out to make a pancake.

The pancake should be cooked for 3 minutes on each side.

Place to a dish, then wrap in plastic wrap to maintain warmth. while you finish the remainder of the pancakes.

Nutritional Information: 182 calories, 13 g fat, 16 g amino, 22 g protein

Glycemic Index: Medium

3.10 Mocha Bowls with Peanut Butter

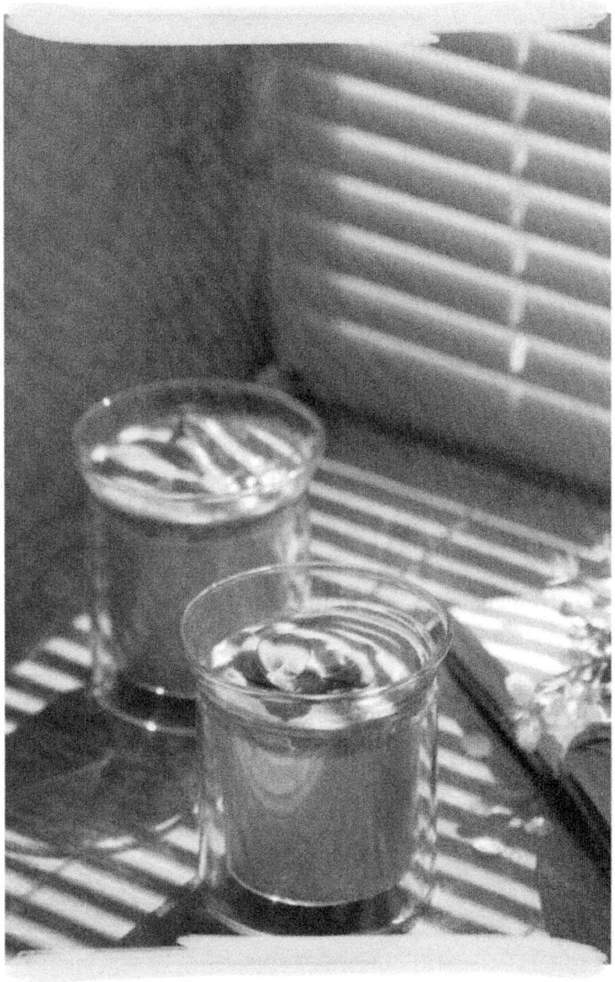

Time spent on preparation: 0 mins

Time spent on cooking: 5 mins

Degree of Difficulty: Easy

Serving: 2

Ingredients:

- 1/3 cup stevia, granulated
- One-third of a cup of cocoa powder
- Cornstarch (2 tbsp.)
- 1 1/2 tea pours coffee granules, instant
- 1 cup half-and-half (fat-free)
- one-quarter cup reduced-fat creamy peanut butter
- Vanilla extract (1/2 tea pour)

Directions:

Combine cornstarch, cocoa powder, stevia, and coffee granules in a moderate saucepan. The heavy cream and half-and-half should be combined in a separate basin. After you reach the highest point of boiling, stir continuously and cook for sixty seconds. Taking the pan off the heat.

In a mixing dish, combine the peanut butter and vanilla extract and whisk until smooth. Fill each of the six dishes with roughly 1/3 cup pudding. Sprinkle extra coffee granules on top of each dish of beaten topping.

Nutritional Information: 271 calories, 13 g fat, 21 g amino, 24 g protein

Glycemic Index: Moderate

3.11 Granola Bars with Cherry and Pecans

Time spent on preparation: 0 mins

Time spent on cooking: 30 mins

Degree of Difficulty: Easy

Serving: 2

Ingredients:

- 2 cups oats, rolled
- 1/2 cup pitted and coarsely chopped dates
- half a cup orange juice
- one quarter cup pecans, chopped
- 1 cup dried fruit-sweetened cherries
- 1/2 teaspoon cinnamon powder
- 1/4 teaspoon allspice powder
- One teaspoon salt, or to taste

Directions:

The oven should now be warmed up to 325 degrees.

On a 13 x 18-inch baking sheet, spread the oats evenly, and bake for ten mins. or until golden brown. Place the oats in a large mixing dish after taking them out of the oven.

Mix in a little pan with the orange juice and dates, and simmer for approximately 15 minutes over moderate-low Warm. Fill a mixer halfway with the ingredients and blend till creamy and smooth.

In a bowl, combine the oats, pecans, dried cherries, cinnamon, allspice, and salt with the date mixture. Completely combine.

Bake the mixture for 20 minutes, or until the top is browned, in an 8-inch nonstick baking pan. Allow cooling completely before cutting into bars.

Nutritional Information: 226 calories, 13 g fat, 11 g amino, 18 g protein

---

3.12 Pumpkin Pudding With Peanut

Time spent on preparation: 10 mins

Time spent on cooking: 60 mins

Degree of Difficulty: Easy

Serving: 2

Ingredients:

- 1/2 a 15-ounce solid pumpkin can
- 1-ounce Pie filling with vanilla instant pudding
- 2 cups half-and-half (fat-free)
- 1/3 cup creamy reduced-fat peanut butter
- One tea pour extract de vanilla
- Two c. fat-free beaten cream

Directions:

In a blender, purée all ingredients, except 1/3 cup of the beaten topping, until smooth. Pour the mixture into six ramekins.

Refrigerate until hard, as directed on the packaging. Serve with the rest of the beaten topping on top.

Nutritional Information: 220 calories, 13 g fat, 16 g amino, 21 g protein

---

3.13 Granola Bars with Almond and Bananas

Time spent on preparation: 10 mins

Time spent on cooking: 25 mins

Degree of Difficulty: Easy

Serving: 2

Ingredients:

- 8 cups oats, rolled
- 2 cups dates, pitted and chopped
- Two peeled and sliced ripe bananas
- One teaspoon of extract (almond)
- One tsp. salt
- One cup almonds

Directions:

To 275 degrees Fahrenheit, rewarm the oven.

Oats should be mixed in a big mixing dish before being set aside. You should line two 13 x 18-inch baking pans with baking paper.

A medium saucepan should contain dates and water (only one cup). For ten minutes, the mixture has to be brought to a gentle simmer. If extra water is needed, add it to prevent the dates from sticking to the pan. Add the banana, almond extract, and salt after removing the liquid from the heat, then purée it in a mixer. Mix the ingredients up until they're smooth and creamy. Well, incorporate the date mixture into the oats. Equilibrate divides the granola between the two prepared pans.

Nutritional Information: 292 calories, 13 g fat, 16 g amino, 24 g protein

CHAPTER 4

SOUP RECIPES

4.1 Miso-Spiced Adzuki Bean Stew

Time spent on preparation: 10 mins

Time spent on cooking: 20 mins

Degree of Difficulty: Easy

Serving: 2

Ingredients:

- One small peeled and sliced big yellow onion
- One medium carrot, peeled and sliced
- Three garlic cloves, peeled and minced
- Two teaspoons of coriander powder
- 2/2 cup soaking adzuki beans
- Two tablespoons miso mellow white
- 1 cup cilantro, chopped
- One teaspoon of red pepper flakes smashed
- season with salt
- eight cups water

Directions:

Carrots and onions should be sautéed for eight minutes over medium heat in a big saucepan. In order to keep the veggies from sticking to the pan, one to two teaspoons of water should be added. using garlic and coriander should be sautéed for an additional minute.

Bring the beans and water in a big saucepan to a boil.

When the beans are tender, place a lid on the pot and simmer for an hour.

Stir mixture until the miso is completely dissolved, then pour it into the saucepan —season with salt, cilantro, and smashed red pepper flakes.

Nutritional Information: 179 calories, 8 g fat, 10 g amino, 7 g protein

4.2 Salmon Soup

Time spent on preparation: 10 mins

Time spent on cooking: 10 mins

Degree of Difficulty: Easy

Serving: 2

Ingredients:

- A spoonful of coconut or avocado oil
- 1/4 cup of red onions that have been finely sliced
- Two tablespoons minced garlic
- 1 pound skinned salmon fillets

- One large tomato, seeded and coarsely chopped
- One tablespoon of fish sauce
- One quarter a teaspoon of acceptable sea salt
- Three cups broth (chicken bone)
- tablespoons chopped fresh dill
- Fresh dill sprigs, capers, sliced fresh chives (optional)

Directions:

Warm the oil in a skillet over a moderate temperature. Combine garlic and onion, then sautè for four mins., stirring until they are fragrant.

In a basin, combine together fresh fish, tomato, salt, fish sauce (if using), and broth. Cook for 12 minutes, or until the salmon is thoroughly cooked, after bringing to a boil over high Heating. Fresh dill sprigs, capers, chives (if used), and freshly ground pepper should be sprinkled on top and served right away.

Nutritional Information: 179 calories, 8 g fat, 10 g amino, 7 g protein

---

4.3 Egyptian Bean Soup

Time spent on preparation: 10 mins

Time spent on cooking: 10 mins

Degree of Difficulty: Easy

Serving: 2

Ingredients:

- One big peeled and chopped yellow onion
- One medium peeled and sliced carrot
- One finely chopped celery stalk
- Four garlic cloves, peeled
- Two tablespoons toasted and ground cumin seeds
- One tablespoon of paprika (sweet)
- bay leaves (two)
- One coarsely sliced big tomato
- 6 cups vegetable stock
- 3 cups fava beans, cooked
- 1/4 teaspoon cayenne pepper
- Two teaspoons mint, finely chopped
- season with salt

Directions:

The onion, carrot, and celery should be sautéed for 10 minutes at medium heat in a large pot. 1-2 tablespoons of water can be added to prevent the vegetables from sticking to the pan. After adding the tomato, bay leaves, garlic, cumin, and paprika, cook for 5 minutes.

Cook fava beans in the vegetable stock for twenty minutes.

Combine cayenne, parsley, mint, inside a large mixing basin. Add salt and simmer for an additional five minutes.

Nutritional Information: 192 calories, 8 g fat, 10 g amino, 7 g protein

---

4.4 Creamy Asparagus Soup

Time spent on preparation: 10 mins

Time spent on cooking: 10 mins

Degree of Difficulty: Easy

Serving: 2

Ingredients:

- One big peeled and chopped yellow onion
- Thyme, 2 tbsp.
- One tablespoon tarragon, chopped
- 4 cups vegetable stock

Directions:

Over medium heat, sauté the onion for 10 minutes in a large saucepan. To prevent the onion from sticking to the pan, add a teaspoon or two of water.

The asparagus, thyme, tarragon, vegetable stock, should be cooked for 20 to 25 minutes, or until the asparagus is extremely tender.

Use a blender or mixer with a tight-fitting cover to gradually puree the soup and a cloth—salt & pepper to taste.

Nutritional Information: 194 calories, 8 g fat, 10 g amino, 7 g protein

4.5 Thai Red Curry Shrimp Soup

Time spent on preparation: 10 mins

Time spent on cooking: 20 mins

Degree of Difficulty: Easy

Serving: 2

Ingredients:

- One tablespoon of avocado oil or coconut oil
- One pound of peeled and deveined medium shrimp
- Fine sea salt and ground black pepper
- Three shallots, finely diced
- 1 1/2 cups of homemade or purchased chicken bone broth
- One can of full-fat coconut milk
- 1 1/2 portions of red curry paste
- 1/4 cup fresh cilantro leaves
- 1/4 cup scallion pieces (about 12 inches long)
- One lime juice slice of lime

Directions:

Warm the oil in a large cast-iron pan over a moderate temperature. The shrimp should be heated for 2 minutes, or until thoroughly cooked, after seasoning with salt and pepper. Take the pan out of the Warm setting and set it aside.

The shallots should be cooked for a further 2 minutes or until tender. Move the fire knob from High to Warm. In a mixing bowl, combine the broth, coconut milk, and curry paste. Stir often while simmering, uncovered, for 10 minutes or until the soup has substantially reduced. The sauce will become thicker the longer you let it simmer.

Mix thoroughly before adding the lime juice, cilantro, and scallions. Add the shrimp to the pan, turn them over, and coat them with sauce. Spoon the soup onto the plates as soon as you remove the pan from the Warm setting. As a garnish, there are lime wedges, cilantro leaves, and sliced scallions.

Nutritional Information: 292 calories, 13 g fat, 16 g amino, 24 g protein

---

4.6 White Beans and Mushroom Stew

Time spent on preparation: 10 mins

Time spent on cooking: 10 mins

Degree of Difficulty: Easy

Serving: 2

Ingredients:

- One moderate peeled and sliced onion

· 1 pound halved cremini mushrooms

· Six garlic cloves, peeled and cut

· One can of chopped tomatoes (14 oz.)

· 14 cup basil, minced

· One tablespoon of thyme, chopped

· teaspoons rosemary, minced

· One leaf of bay

· 2 sautéed navy beans in cups (drained and rinsed)

Directions:

In a big saucepan, sauté the onion and mushrooms for 10 minutes over moderate temperature. To prevent the vegetables from sticking to the pan, add 1 to 2 tablespoons of water. Add the garlic and cook for one minute.

On high heat, bring the pot to a boil. Stirring the tomatoes, basil, thyme, rosemary, bay leaf, and beans.

Reduce the temperature to moderate-low and cook for 15 minutes, covered.

Nutritional Information: 179 calories, 8 g fat, 10 g amino, 7 g protein

---

4.7 Orzo & Turkey Soup

Time spent on preparation: 10 mins

Time spent on cooking: 10 mins

Degree of Difficulty: Easy

Serving: 2

Ingredients:

- Two tablespoons of coconut oil
- Three tablespoons finely diced onions
- 2 cups roughly chopped cauliflower florets
- 6 cups homemade or store-bought chicken bone broth
- 1 1/2 cups sliced roasted turkey or chicken
- Fine sea salt (optional) 3 teaspoons chopped fresh dill, plus extra for garnish

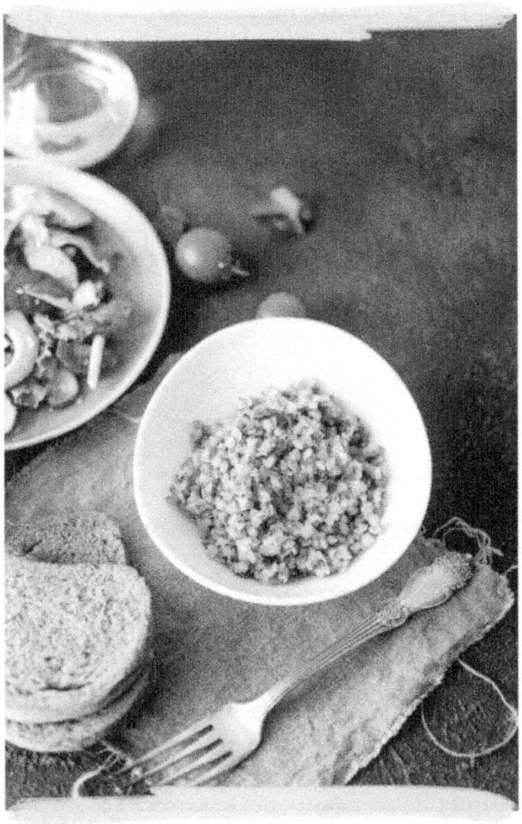

Directions:

In a Dutch oven or stockpot, heat the coconut oil until it has completely melted.

The onions should be translucent after 4 minutes of sautéing. Fry the cauliflower for a further three minutes. Until the stock, turkey, and dill are fully cooked, simmer for 3 minutes—taste, and if required, season with salt.

Nutritional Information: 292 calories, 13 g fat, 16 g amino, 24 g protein

4.8 Basic Chili Stew

Time spent on preparation: 10 mins

Time spent on cooking: 20 mins

Degree of Difficulty: Easy

Serving: 2

Ingredients:

- One small peeled and sliced medium yellow onion
- Two garlic cloves, peeled and minced
- 2 tbsp. ginger, grated
- 2 tsp. Thai red chilli paste
- One lime, zest and juice
- 1 minced Serrano chili
- Two tablespoons of soy sauce
- One light coconut milk can (14 oz.)
- 1 cup vegetable stock
- 3 cups mixed veggies
- 1/2 cup cilantro, chopped
- 2 tbsp. mint (minced)

Directions:

In a medium skillet, fry the onions for 7 to 8 minutes over a moderate flame or until they are soft and beginning to caramelize. Add 1 to 2 teaspoons of water to prevent the onions from clinging to the pan.

After incorporating the garlic, ginger, and chilli paste, lime zest and juice, and Serrano chilli.

Reduce the heat to medium, Simmer for 10 minutes, or until the vegetables are tender, adding the soy sauce, coconut milk, vegetable stock, and mixed vegetables. a garnish of cilantro and mint on top.

Nutritional Information: 292 calories, 13 g fat, 16 g amino, 24 g protein

---

4.9 Red Pepper & Tomato Soup

Time spent on preparation: 10 mins

Time spent on cooking: 10 mins

Degree of Difficulty: Easy

Serving: 2

Ingredients:

- Two medium peeled and roughly chopped yellow onions
- Two seeded and finely chopped big red bell peppers
- Three big peeled and chopped garlic cloves
- 1 tbsp. dried leaves of thyme
- 1 pound roughly chopped fresh tomatoes (about three medium)
- 1/4 cup chiffonier basil

Directions:

The onions and red pepper should be cooked for ten minutes at medium heat in a big skillet. 1-2 tablespoons of water can be added to prevent the vegetables from sticking to the pan.

Add the tomatoes and simmer for 20 minutes with the lid on after adding the garlic and thyme. Process the soup in stages in an electric mixer or food processor with a tight-fitting lid and a towel covering it.

Nutritional Information: 179 calories, 8 g fat, 10 g amino, 7 g protein

---

4.10 Coconut Ginger Chicken Soup

Time spent on preparation: 10 mins

Time spent on cooking: 20 mins

Degree of Difficulty: Easy

Serving: 2

Ingredients:

- 4 cups full-fat coconut milk
- 1/4 cup peeled and grated fresh ginger
- garlic cloves, chopped
- stalks lemongrass

- sliced three shallots
- chopped one teaspoon
- crushed white pepper
- boneless, skinless chicken breast halves
- 1/2 teaspoon fine sea salt
- Two limes, grated zest
- Three tablespoons of fish sauce
- Serrano chili peppers, chopped

Directions:

Prepare the ginger paste by pulsing or pounding the ginger and garlic in a stick blender or mortar (using the pestle). Pulverize the lemongrass, shallots, and white pepper. Remove from the equation.

Bring the coconut milk to a boil in a medium saucepan. If you overcook it, it will curdle. Stir in the ginger paste, then bring to a boil the mixture to a boil while adding the chicken. Combine lime zest, fish sauce, chilies, and salt in a mixing bowl. Cover and cook for 45 minutes over medium-low Warm or until the chicken is thoroughly cooked.

Nutritional Information: 292 calories, 13 g fat, 16 g amino, 24 g protein

---

4.11 Thai-Noodle Soup

Time spent on preparation: 10 mins

Time spent on cooking: 10 mins

Degree of Difficulty: Easy

Serving: 2

Ingredients:

- One medium peeled and thinly sliced yellow onion
- One medium peeled and julienned carrot
- 6 oz. shiitake mushrooms (without stems)
- Three garlic cloves, peeled and minced
- One tablespoon ginger, grated
- 2 cups bok Choy, sliced
- 4 cups vegetable stock
- 2 tbsp. soy sauce (low sodium)
- One lime, zest, and juice
- 1 Serrano chili, stemmed and thinly sliced
- 6 oz. brown rice noodles, cooked
- 1 cup sprouted mung beans
- 12 cup cilantro, chopped

Directions:

The mushrooms, onion, and carrot should be sautéed for 7 to 8 minutes in a medium pot.

To stop the veggies from sticking to the pan, add one to two teaspoons of water. Lime zest, lime juice, Serrano chile, garlic, ginger, bok choy, vegetable stock, and soy sauce are added to the pan. Using a high heat, bring to a boil. Cook for a further 10 minutes with the heat set to medium-low.

Nutritional Information: 292 calories, 13 g fat, 16

g amino, 24 g protein

4.12 Chilled Tomatoes & Ham Soup

Time spent on preparation: 10 mins

Time spent on cooking: 20 mins

Degree of Difficulty: Easy

Serving: 2

Ingredients:

- 3/4 pound plum tomatoes, quartered
- One garlic clove
- 1/4 cup avocado oil
- One tablespoon of coconut vinegar
- Fine sea salt
- powdered black pepper
- 4 thin slices prosciutto

Directions:

Tomatoes, garlic, and other ingredients should be blended or processed in a food smooth. Refrigerate for approximately 15 minutes, until cool, after seasoning with salt and pepper.

To serve, spoon cold soup into bowls and sprinkle with vinegar and oil. Serve the soup with ham slices. If desired, garnish with fresh herbs.

Keep up it for three days in an airtight jar. Nutritional Information: 292 calories, 13 g fat, 16 g amino, 24 g protein

---

CHAPTER 5

SALADS AND SIDES RECIPES

5.1 Asian Vegetable Salad

Time spent on preparation: 5 mins

Time spent on cooking: 20 mins

Degree of Difficulty: Easy

Serving: 2

Ingredients:

- Four limes, one lime zest, and two lime juice
- 1/4 cup rice syrup (brown)
- Soy sauce
- Two tablespoons of rice vinegar (brown)
- 4 cups Napa cabbage, finely chopped
- One seeded and julienned red bell pepper
- One bunch of green onions
- 1 cup sprouted mung beans
- 1/2 cup cilantro, chopped
- 1/2 cup basil leaves, chopped
- 1 Serrano chili, thinly cut on the diagonal (remove the seeds for reduced heat)
- Two teaspoons mint, chopped

Directions:

In a large mixing bowl, combine the lime zest and juice, brown rice syrup, and soy sauce (if using).

In a separate bowl, toss the cabbage, brown rice vinegar, mung beans, onion, spices, and aromatic herbs.

Ponzu Sauce should be served alongside.

Nutritional Information: 251 calories, 13 g fat, 16 g amino, 24 g protein

---

5.2 Lentils & Fresh Herb Salad

Time spent on preparation: 5 mins

Time spent on cooking: 20 mins

Degree of Difficulty: Easy

Serving: 2

Ingredients:

- Half cup washed green lentils
- Three mugs of vegetable broth or vegetable stock
- One lemon's zest and two lemons' juice
- Two onion, one of which finely sliced for garnish
- Half cup cilantro, finely chopped
- Two teaspoons mint, finely chopped
- arugula, 4 cups

Directions:

Lentils and vegetable stock should be combined and heated over medium heat until they are boiling. Decrease the heat to low, cover the pot, and simmer the lentils for 35 to 45 minutes, or until they are tender but not mushy.

After rinsing the lentils, put them in a large mixing bowl. Add the green onion, cilantro, mint, lemon zest, juice, and season with salt and pepper.

Divide the arugula among four separate dishes to serve. Serve the lentil salad over the greens, topped with finely sliced green onion.

Nutritional Information: 361 calories, 13 g fat, 16 g amino, 24 g protein

---

5.3 Wheat Berries Salad

Time spent on preparation: 10 mins

Time spent on cooking: 20 mins

Degree of Difficulty: Easy

Serving: 2

Ingredients:

- 2 1/2 cups wheat berries
- 1/4 cup apple cider vinegar plus two teaspoons
- 1/4 cup rice syrup (brown)
- 1/2 cup minced green onion
- Two celery stalks
- Two teaspoons of tarragon, minced
- One cored and diced Bosc pear
- 1/2 cup dried cranberries, sweetened with fruit

Directions:

Five cups of water should be boiled in a medium saucepan before adding the wheat berries. Bring the mixture back to a boil over high heat.

After the wheat berries are tender, decrease the heat to medium, cover the pot, and simmer it for one hour.

After being cleaned, the berries should be taken out of the pan and refrigerated.

In a large basin, mix the remaining ingredients. Add the wheat berries then. Chill for one hour before serving.

Nutritional Information: 217 calories, 13 g fat, 16 g amino, 24 g protein

---

5.4 Tomato, Cucumber and Mint Salad

Time spent on preparation: 10 mins

Time spent on cooking: 20 mins

Degree of Difficulty: Easy

Serving: 2

Ingredients:

- 1/4 cup balsamic vinegar

- Two big tomatoes, diced
- Two big cucumbers
- diced two green onions
- Two tablespoons mint, finely chopped
- Spices (salt, pepper)

Directions:

Using a cutting board and a knife you will have to clean and cut all the vegetables. As soon as you have finished you can prepare your salad.

You are going to place the already cleaned and sliced vegetables inside a salad bowl, then season them with spices and balsamic vinegar.

Allow 30 minutes to sit before serving.

Nutritional Information: 231 calories, 13 g fat, 16 g amino, 24 g protein

---

5.5 Grains Salad

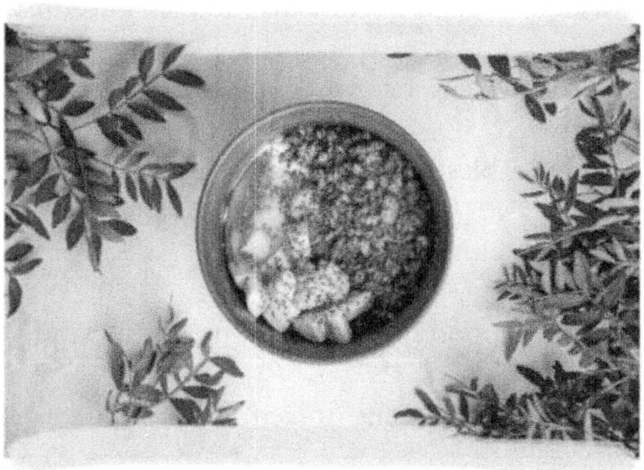

Time spent on preparation: 0 mins

Time spent on cooking: 10 mins

Degree of Difficulty: Easy

Serving: 2

Ingredients:

- 2 cups of brown basmati rice
- Two limes, juice, and zest
- 1/4 cup of each brown rice syrup and brown rice vinegar
- a cup of currants
- 1/2 tiny red onion, peeled and minced
- Six green onions, coarsely chopped
- One minced jalapeno pepper
- curry powder (about one tablespoon)
- 1/4 cup cilantro, chopped

Directions:

Rinse the rice in cold water and then strain it. In a saucepan, combine it with 4 cups of cold water. After the rice is tender, after about 45 to 50 minutes of boiling at high heat, decrease the heat to moderate. Soft.

Combine the currants, green onion, red onion, jalapeno pepper, curry powder, cilantro, salt, and pepper in a large mixing bowl along with the lime zest and juice while the rice is cooking.

Removed rice from the water should be put to the mixing bowl and well combined with rice syrup and vinegar.

Nutritional Information: 189 calories, 13 g fat, 16 g

amino, 24 g protein

5.6 Argula & Quinoa Salad

Time spent on preparation: 10 mins

Time spent on cooking: 10 mins

Degree of Difficulty: Easy

Serving: 2

Ingredients:

- 1/2 cup quinoa
- One lime and two oranges, zest and juice for each
- 1/4 cup rice vinegar (brown)
- Arugula, 4 cups
- One small peeled red onion
- 1 seeded red bell pepper, cut into 12-inch chunks
- 1 teaspoon toasted pine nuts

Directions:

Drain the quinoa after washing it in cold water. In a saucepan, bring 3 cups of water to a boil.

With the quinoa added, return the water to a boil over high heat.

Once the quinoa has finished cooking, turn the heat down to medium-low, cover the pot, and let it simmer for 15 to 20 minutes.

On a baking sheet, the quinoa should be dried and allowed to cool.

In a sizable mixing bowl, combine the arugula, onion, red pepper, pine nuts, brown rice vinegar, orange, and lime zest and juice as the quinoa cools. Once the quinoa has cooled, add it and chill for an hour before serving.

Nutritional Information: 197 calories, 13 g fat, 16 g amino, 24 g protein

---

5.7 Beats, Beans & Orange Salad

Time spent on preparation: 10 mins

Time spent on cooking: 10 mins

Degree of Difficulty: Easy

Serving: 2

Ingredients:

- Five medium beets, cleaned and peeled
- Two oranges, (fruit and zest already peeled and cutted
- 2 cups cooked navy beans (drained and rinsed)
- A quarter cup rice vinegar (brown)
- Three tablespoons dill, minced
- season with salt to taste
- 1/2 teaspoon black pepper, freshly ground
- 4 cups salad greens (mixed)

Directions:

In a saucepan with some water still in it, beets are

added. Beets should be simmered for 20 minutes or until soft after coming to a boil, so reduce the heat to medium.

Beets should be taken out of the water and set aside to cool.

Cut the chilled beets into wedges, and then put them in a large mixing bowl.

With the beans, dill, salt, pepper, brown rice vinegar, orange zest, and segments, flip the beets. Gently flip to combine.

To serve, divide the mixed salad greens into four different bowls.

Nutritional Information: 173 calories, 13 g fat, 16 g amino, 24 g protein

---

5.8 Chicken & Grape Salad

Time spent on preparation: 10 mins

Time spent on cooking: 10 mins

Degree of Difficulty: Easy

Serving: 2

Ingredients:

· 1/2 cup diced celery

· Ten grapes

· 1/4 cup slivered almonds

· tablespoons poppy seeds

· One tablespoon of chopped fresh dill

· One tablespoon of dry mustard

· Six boneless, skinless chicken breasts

· tablespoons olive oil

Directions:

Fill a stockpot halfway with water and add the chicken breasts.

After bringing to a boil, lower heat to a low Warm and simmer until the chicken is fully cooked—approximately 20 minutes. Drain.

Combine the chicken and olive oil in a blender or food processor. Pulse the chicken until it is finely chopped.

Flip the chicken with the celery, grapes (if using), almonds, poppy seeds, dill, and mustard in a large mixing dish. Serve right away, or cover and chill for up to a week.

Nutritional Information: 162 calories, 13 g fat, 16 g amino, 24 g protein

---

5.9 Succotash Salad

Time spent on preparation: 0 mins

Time spent on cooking: 5 mins

Degree of Difficulty: Easy

Serving: 2

Ingredients:

· 1/2 cup baby lima beans, cooked

· Three corn ears

· 1/4 cup balsamic vinegar

· 1/4 cup chopped parsley

· Two big tomatoes, chopped

· One medium red onion, peeled and sliced

Directions:

Unite everything in a large bowl and give it a good toss.

Nutritional Information: 166 calories, 13 g fat, 16 g amino, 24 g protein

---

5.10 Wedge Salad with Ranch Dressing

Time spent on preparation: 10 mins

Time spent on cooking: 10 mins

Degree of Difficulty: Easy

Serving: 2

Ingredients:

· 1/2 cup low-carb, dairy-free ranch dressing

· Six tablespoons of bacon bits

· One tomato, diced

· Four radishes, diced

· 1/4 cup finely minced fresh chives

· 1/2 of a teaspoon of freshly ground black pepper

Directions:

Place the lettuce wedges on four separate serving dishes. 2 tablespoons dressing on top of each wedge; flip in the bacon pieces, tomato, radishes, chives, and salt & pepper to taste. Serve right away.

Nutritional Information: 162 calories, 13 g fat, 16 g amino, 24 g protein

---

5.11 Purple Potatoes & Kale Salad

Time spent on preparation: 10 mins

Time spent on cooking: 10 mins

Degree of Difficulty: Easy

Serving: 2

Ingredients:

- 2 cups chopped kale
- 1/2 cup crushed tomatoes
- Citrus juice
- 1 cup of chopped cilantro
- Two tablespoons of tahini
- Four potatoes
- One garlic clove, peeled and chopped
- One teaspoon cayenne pepper, 1/2 teaspoon salt, or to taste

Directions:

Put the potatoes and just enough water to cover them in a medium saucepan.

Bring to a simmer, reduce heat to medium-low, and simmer for about 10 minutes, or until the kale is tender to the fork. Potatoes are drained and placed aside to cool. After cooled, peel if desired, and cut into 12-inch pieces.

In a pan or skillet, cook the kale and tomatoes until the kale softens, about 2 to 3 minutes somewhat. Add 1 – 2 teaspoons of water to avoid the veggies sticking to the pan. Allow cooling after adding 1/4 teaspoons of lime juice.

Blend the cilantro, garlic, tahini, remaining lime juice, salt, cayenne pepper, and two tablespoons of water together until its smooth. Blend until completely smooth.

Make a bed of cooked kale and tomatoes in a big salad bowl, add boiled potatoes on top, and sprinkle with the dressing to serve.

Nutritional Information: 152 calories, 13 g fat, 16 g amino, 24 g protein

---

5.12 Basic Broccoli Salad

Time spent on preparation: 10 mins

Time spent on cooking: 10 mins

Degree of Difficulty: Easy

Serving: 2

Ingredients:

- One bag broccoli
- low-carb mayonnaise
- Sunflower seeds salted in six tablespoons
- Chopped red onion, 1/2 cup
- 1/4 cup vinegar, white
- Four pieces of Perfect Bacon, chopped (optional)

Directions

Combine the broccoli slaw, mayonnaise, sunflower seeds, onion, vinegar, and bacon in an airtight container (if using).

Wait for at least 2 hours, covered. Allow cooling before serving. Store in the refrigerator in an airtight container for up to three days.

Nutritional Information: 159 calories, 13 g fat, 16 g amino, 24 g protein

CHAPTER 6

MEAT RECIPES

6.1 Skillet Casserole with Ground Beef

Time spent on preparation: 5mins

Time spent on cooking: 45-60mins

Level of Difficulty: Easy

Serving: 2

Ingredients:

- 1 pound of extra-lean · beef (90 percent lean) beef
- 4 oz. rotini (multigrain or whole grain)
- 1 (14.5-ounce) may no longer be used
- stirred tomatoes with salt
- 1 1/2 cups green bell pepper, chopped
- Four oz. mushrooms, sliced
- Ketchup, 1/4 cup
- Worcestershire sauce, one tablespoon
- 1 tbsp. balsamic vinaigrette
- 1 cup of water
- Salt (1/4 teaspoon)

Directions:

Heat up a large nonstick pan on medium-high. For three minutes, flip the meat often while cooking it in batches. Trim the meat of any extra fat.

In a bowl, combine the remaining ingredients. To cook the noodles, after bringing the mixture after which, set the temperature to low, cover the pot, and let it simmer for 15 minutes.

Nutritional Information: 292 calories, 13 g fat, 16 g amino, 24 g protein

---

6.2 Beef Burritos

Time spent on preparation: 10 mins

Time spent on cooking: 30 mins

Level of Difficulty: Easy

Serving: 2

Ingredients:

- 1.5-pound beef chuck pot roast
- Two tablespoons of taco sauce Verde
- Two teaspoons of minced garlic
- One scallion or spring onions, big
- 2 chopped jalapeño peppers
- One teaspoon of cayenne pepper
- 1/4 tsp. Cumin and 1/4 tsp. salt
- Half cup broth

Directions:

Trim away as much fat as possible from the meat.

Combine all the ingredients in a slow cooker, then tighten the cover.

Cook the beef for eight hours or until it is soft.

On a chopping board, place the steak and use a fork and knife to shred it (one to hold the meat and the other to shred it.)

In a serving dish, place the shredded meat.

Pour 1/2 cup of the cooking liquid into the mixing bowl and thoroughly combine.

Nutritional Information: 272 calories, 13 g fat, 16 g amino, 24 g protein

---

6.3 Beef Liver Burgers

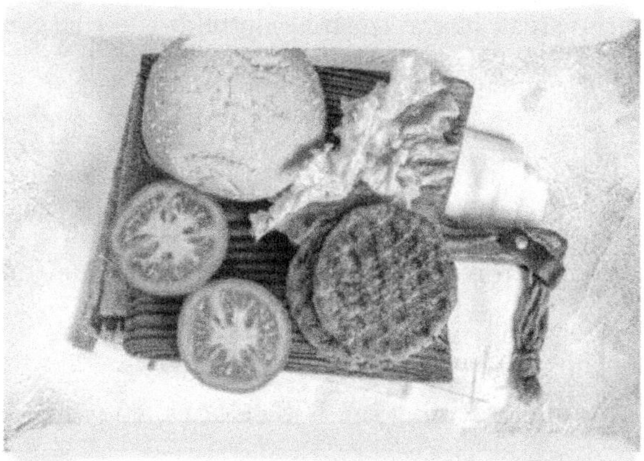

Time spent on preparation: 10 mins

Time spent on cooking: 30 mins

Level of Difficulty: Easy

Serving: 2

Ingredients:

- 1 pound of beef or bison, chopped into tiny pieces
- 8 ounces of beef liver, cut into small pieces
- Three tablespoons of stevia-free ketchup
- Three teaspoons garlic salt, spiced

Directions:

Combine and knead the ground beef,

liver, ketchup, in a small bowl with two teaspoons of garlic salt. Make 4 to 6 burger patties from the mixture.

Over medium heat, warm the oil in a cast iron skillet. On top of the burgers, add the final teaspoon of garlic salt. Cook until well done, about 8 to 10 minutes per side.

Nutritional Information: 264 calories, 13 g fat, 16 g amino, 24 g protein

---

6.4 Beef with Sesame Sauce

Time spent on preparation: 10 mins

Time spent on cooking: 40 mins

Level of Difficulty: Easy

Serving: 2

Ingredients:

- 30 ml or one-fourth cup of extra virgin olive oil
- a quarter cup (26 g) of stevia

- a quarter cup (30 ml) of Soy Sauce
- Two garlic cloves of garlic
- a quarter cup (25 g) of green onions, chopped
- to taste black pepper
- 1 pound (455 g) cut-in-strips round steak
- One tablespoon (8 g) of roasted sesame seeds
- Rice already cooked

Directions:

Mix one tablespoon (15 ml) of oil, stevia, soy sauce, garlic, green onions, and pepper in a mixing bowl. Marinate the meat for at least 20 minutes in this compound.

Heat the remaining oil in a skillet or wok. Stir-fry the meat with the marinade. Serve with rice and sesame seeds on top.

Nutritional Information: 239 calories, 13 g fat, 16 g amino, 24 g protein

---

6.5 Sweet Soy Flank

Time spent on preparation: 10 mins

Time spent on cooking: 45 mins

Level of Difficulty: Easy

Serving: 2

Ingredients:

- 1/4 cup soy sauce (mild)
- Ketchup, two tablespoons
- 1 tbsp. balsamic vinaigrette
- 1/4 teaspoon of garlic powder
- Half a teaspoon powdered onion
- 1/4 teaspoon pepper flakes (dry)
- Flank steak, 1 1/2 pound
- Two tablespoons green onion, finely chopped (optional)

Directions:

Mix all ingredients (excluding green onion) in a gallon-size plastic bag, close firmly, and flip back and forth until thoroughly mixed. Refrigerate for up to 48 hours, but no less than 8 hours.

Preheat the grill pan to medium-high. Spray the grill pan with nonstick cooking spray.

Put the steak in the trash along with the marinade. To dry the steak, use paper towels. Cook for four minutes on each side. (Note: if you continue to boil it, it will turn tough.) Put the meat on a chopping board and set aside for 10 minutes before slicing it thinly across the grain.

Nutritional Information: 350 calories, 13 g fat, 16 g amino, 24 g protein

---

6.6 Beef with Rice Noodles

Time spent on preparation: 10 mins

Time spent on cooking: 45 mins

Level of Difficulty: Moderate

Serving: 2

Ingredients:

- Boneless beef round steak, 13/4 pound (795 g)
- Four tablespoons sake or sherry (60 ml) split
- One tablespoon of oil (6 g) of ginger root, finely chopped
- Three tablespoons vegetable oil (45 ml), divided
- 4 ounces (115 g) rice noodles, one garlic clove, smashed
- 2 cups thinly sliced bok Choy
- thinly sliced green olives

Directions:

Trim any excess fat from the beef steak. Cut the meat into 1/4-inch (5 mm) strips diagonally. Mix the meat, two tablespoons (30 ml) sake, gingerroot, two teaspoons (10 ml) oil, and garlic in a medium glass or plastic bowl.

Thirty minutes after covering, place in the fridge. Place the rice noodles in a large mixing bowl. Boiling water should be placed halfway up the container. Ten minutes of waiting should be given before full draining. Chop the veggies roughly.

Heat one teaspoon of oil in a wok. For approximately 5 minutes, or until the beef is well cooked, the meat mixture should be stirred.

In a large mixing bowl, combine the rice noodles, bok Choy, and onions. Bok choy should be cooked for 4 minutes or until crisp-tender.

Nutritional Information: 292 calories, 13 g fat, 16 g amino, 24 g protein

---

6.7 Quiche Tacos

Time spent on preparation: 10mins

Time spent on cooking: 45 - 65mins

Level of Difficulty: Easy

Serving: 2

Ingredients:

- Extra-lean beef ground up
- Taco seasoning, 2 tbsp. (8 g)
- water, 1/2 cup (120 ml)
- 1/2 cup (58 g) low-fat shredded cheese
- 2 ounces (55 g) of chopped green chillies, seeded
- three eggs
- 1 cup fat-free evaporated milk (235 mL)

Directions:

After turning on the oven, reach the temperature of 370° Fahrenheit. In a skillet, brown the meat. Add the water and taco seasoning mix, and stir. Then while covered, permit chilling for ten minutes.

Mix in the cheese and chillies well. Fill a pie pan with the mixture after spraying it with nonstick vegetable oil.

Mix eggs and milk in a mixing bowl. Blend until completely smooth. Bake for forty-five minutes in a preheated oven, or until custard is set.

Before serving, let the pie five minutes to rest.

Nutritional Information: 262 calories, 13 g fat, 16 g amino, 24 g protein

---

6.8 Ground Beef and Cabbage Slaw

Time spent on preparation: 10 mins

Time spent on cooking: 30 mins

Level of Difficulty: Easy

Serving: 2

Ingredients:

- 1 pound of beef, ground
- 1 (16-ounce) bag cabbage slaw mix
- Three tablespoons of coconut aminos
- One tablespoon of fish sauce

Directions:

In a large pan, the olive oil should be heated at a medium-high temperature. Cook for about 7 minutes, turning the meat once in a while until browned. Cook for about 15 minutes, regularly tossing the cabbage, until it has wilted.

After including the coconut aminos and fish sauce, cook for an additional five minutes.

Nutritional Information: 299 calories, 13 g fat, 15 g amino, 21 g protein

---

6.9 Easy-to-make Meatloaf

Time spent on preparation: 10mins

Time spent on cooking: 15mins

Level of Difficulty: Easy Serving: 2

Ingredients:

- 12 oz. extra-lean beef (90 percent lean) beef in the ground
- 1/2 cup oats (quick-cooking)
- 1 (14-ounce) container of thawed frozen pepper stir-fry
- A quarter cup of egg repayment
- One teaspoon of oregano leaves, dried
- Pizza sauce (about 3/4 cup)
- 1 tbsp. Parmesan cheese, grated (optional)

Directions:

Preheat the oven to 350 degrees Fahrenheit. Add the meat, oats, stir fry, egg, oregano, and all but 1/4 cup of the pizza sauce in a medium mixing basin.

Pour the batter into the pan that has been sprayed with spray oil.

Bake for one hour, or until a meat thermometer reads 160°F when using a baking dish. Spread the remaining pizza sauce equally over the top and top with cheese (if preferred). Slice into eight pieces after waiting five minutes.

Nutritional Information: 292 calories, 13 g fat, 16 g amino, 24 g protein

---

6.10 Bleu Patty Burger

Time spent on preparation: 10 mins

Time spent on cooking: 10 mins

Level of Difficulty: Easy

Serving: 2

Ingredients:

- Burger patty Bleu Burger, pound (150 g)
- g blue cheese crumbles
- 1 tbsp. sweet red onion (finely chopped)

Directions:

Using your favorite technique, cook the burger. Top with the bleu cheese and let it melt when it's nearly done to your preference.

The pan should be taken from the heat, put on a plate, and topped with the onion..

Nutritional Information: 248 calories, 13 g fat, 16 g amino, 24 g protein

Glycemic Index: Moderate

6.11 Greek Goulash

Time spent on preparation: 10 mins

Time spent on cooking: 45-60 mins

Level of Difficulty: Easy

Serving: 2

Ingredients:

- 350 g peeled shallots
- 2-3 cloves of peeled garlic
- Carrots, 2
- 4 tbsp. extra virgin olive oil
- 550 g beef goulash
- salt and pepper
- 125 ml red wine
- ½ bunch of oregano
- cinnamon sticks
- bay leaves
- 1 pinch each of nutmeg and cumin
- 200 g tomato puree

- 600 mL stock (meat)
- 6 tbsp. thickener for the dark sauce

Directions:

Peel and cut shallots in half. Garlic should also be peeled and coarsely chopped. Peel the carrots and cut them into small pieces.

In a casserole, heat the olive oil and cook the goulash. Add the shallots, garlic, and carrots to the pan and cook until softened. Season with salt and pepper and deglaze with red wine.

Wash the oregano, and combine it in a mixing dish with the meat, bay leaves, and cinnamon. Nutmeg and cumin are used as seasonings. Toss in the tomatoes and beef stock.

Cover and bake for about 1-2 hours at 180 degrees (convection: 160 degrees) in a preheated oven. Stir in the the\sauce thickener and simmer for 1 minute.

Apply salt and pepper to season once more. Finally, if desired, serve with Greek rice noodles.

Nutritional Information: 285 calories, 13 g fat, 16 g amino, 24 g protein

---

6.12 Spicy Ground Beef with Almonds

Time spent on preparation: 10 mins

Time spent on cooking: 25 mins

Level of Difficulty: Easy

Serving: 2

Ingredients:

- 10 oz. extra-lean ground beef
- 1 cup yellow onion, chopped
- One medium red bell pepper
- eggplant cubes
- 1/4 cup raisins (dark)
- 1/2 tablespoons allspice powder
- One teaspoon of cumin powder
- 1 ounce slivered almonds, toasted if possible
- A half teaspoon of salt
- 1 cup fresh mint, chopped and divided
- 1/2 cup plain Greek yogurt (nonfat)

Directions:

Preheat medium-high heat in a big nonstick skillet. Brown the meat in a skillet. Remove any excess fat. Mix the onions, bell pepper, eggplant, raisins, allspice, and cumin in a big bowl. The onions should be extremely soft after 30 minutes of simmering.

Mix the almonds, salt, and all rest but two tablespoons of the mint in a mixing bowl.

Nutritional Information: 292 calories, 13 g fat, 16 g amino, 24 g protein

---

Chapter 7

VEGETARIAN AND VEGAN RECIPES

7.1 Acorn Squash with Stuffing

Time spent on preparation: 10mins

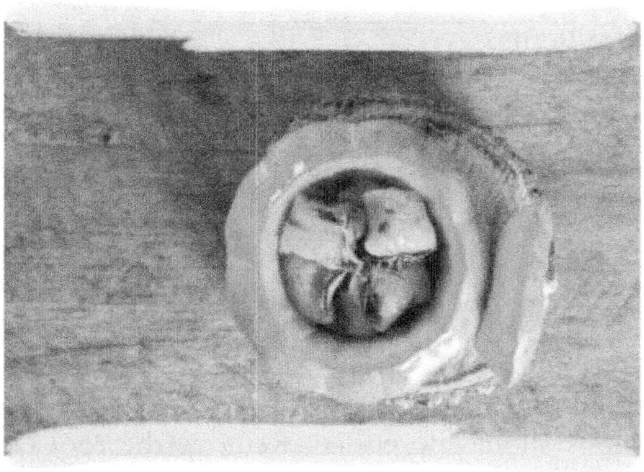

Time spent on cooking: 10mins

Level of Difficulty: Easy

Serving: 2

Ingredients:

- Squash acorns
- Two peeled and chopped apples
- 1/2 cup brown stevia
- A quarter teaspoon of cinnamon
- Nutmeg (1/4 teaspoon)
- Lemon juice, two tablespoons
- 1/4 cup unsalted butter

Directions:

Take the apple, split it lengthwise in half, then take out all the seeds. Evenly distribute the diced apple among the squash halves.

Sprinkle a quarter of the brown stevia, cinnamon, nutmeg, and a few drops of lemon juice over each half. One tablespoon (14 g) butter, a dot on each. Wrap each squash half in foil tightly.

Fill the slow cooker with 14 cups (60 milliliters) of water. Stack the squash in the cooker, and cut the side up. Cook on low for 5 hours, covered. Unwrap the squash and arrange it on a serving plate.

Nutritional Information: 168 calories, 10 g fat, 13 g amino, 11 g protein

---

7.2 Mussels Steamed in Coconut Broth

Time spent on preparation: 10mins

Time spent on cooking: 10mins

Level of Difficulty: Easy

Serving: 2

Ingredients:

- 2 tbsp. of unsalted butter
- 1 cup chopped shallots
- Minced garlic cloves
- Two teaspoons of seasoning (Italian)
- 1 tbsp. stevia extract
- 1 cup tomatoes, cherry

- mussels, 2 lbs., cleaned and rinsed
- 1 quart of coconut milk
- 1 tbsp. tapioca flour

Directions:

In the Instant Pot, melt the butter in the sauté mode.

Sauté the shallots until they are soft. (approximately 2 minutes)

Add the garlic, stir, and cook until fragrant. (approximately 1 minute.)

Cook after adding the cherry tomatoes, constantly stirring, until the sauce boils.

Return to a boil with the remaining ingredients (excluding the finishing ingredients).

Add the mussels and stir until everything is well mixed.

Close and lock the lid.

Change the vent's setting to Sealing.

Cook for 6 minutes under high pressure.

In a small dish, mix the coconut milk and tapioca starch.

Pour the milk mixture into the Instant Pot until the soup thickens.

Nutritional Information: 163 calories, 10 g fat, 13 g amino, 11 g protein

---

7.3 Caramelized Onions

Time spent on preparation: 10mins

Time spent on cooking: 10mins

Level of Difficulty: Easy

Serving: 2

Ingredients:

- Six big sweet onions
- 1/4 cup (55 g) butter
- 1/4 cup (285 ml) chicken broth

Directions:

Onions should be peeled. Remove the root ends and stems. Put everything in the slow cooker.

Butter and broth should be poured over the onions. Cook for 12 hours on low.

Nutritional Information: 162 calories, 10 g fat, 13 g amino, 11 g protein

7.4 Italian-Style Stuffed Tomatoes

Time spent on preparation: 10mins

Time spent on cooking: 10mins

Level of Difficulty: Easy

Serving: 2

Ingredients:

- Four mugs of navy beans, once cooked (drained and rinsed)
- 1/2 moderate yellow onion, peeled and sliced into tiny
- artichoke hearts (oil-free), drained and

coarsely chopped

- Six big tomatoes (beefsteak, for example)

Directions:

Combine the beans, artichoke hearts, onion, and pesto. and mix; put aside.

Slice each tomato's top in half, removing the flesh and leaving a 12-inch shell.

Nutritional Information: 161 calories, 10 g fat, 13 g amino, 11 g protein

---

7.5 Greek Green Beans & Tomatoes

Time spent on preparation: 10mins

Time spent on cooking: 10mins

Level of Difficulty: Easy

Serving: 2

Ingredients:

- Fresh green beans, 1 pound
- One mug (235 ml) of chopped tomatoes with no salt added
- One mug (160 g) onion, chopped
- 1/2 teaspoon oregano, dry
- 1 tsp. lemon extract
- One tablespoon (15 ml) of extra virgin olive oil
- To taste black pepper

Directions:

Stir all of the ingredients together in a slow cooker. Stir. Cook covered on low for six hours.

Nutritional Information: 188 calories, 10 g fat, 13 g amino, 11 g protein

---

7.6 Orange Flavored Carrots

Time spent on preparation: 10mins

Time spent on cooking: 15mins

Level of Difficulty: Easy

Serving: 2

Ingredients:

- quarts liquid
- 1 pound peeled and sliced carrots
- 1 1/2 tablespoons orange zest, grated
- tbsp. reduced-fat (50 percent vegetable oil) spread like margarine
- 2 tbsp. dark brown stevia, packed
- One teaspoon of mustard (Dijon)
- Salt (1/4 teaspoon)

Directions:

Fill a big saucepan halfway with water. In a saucepan, place the foldable steamer basket.

Carrots should be arranged in a basket. On high heat, bring to a boil while coated. Sauté the carrots for 8 minutes or until they are soft and crisp.

Take off the carrots out of the steamer basket and mix them with the other ingredients in a moderate mixing dish.

Nutritional Information: 296 calories, 13 g fat, 16 g amino, 24 g protein

---

7.7 Basic Lima Beans

Time spent on preparation: 10mins

Time spent on cooking: 10mins

Level of Difficulty: Easy

Serving: 2

Ingredients:

Dried lima beans, 1 · pound (455 g)

· 12 cups chopped onion (240 g)

· 12 cup celery, chopped (50 g)

· big peeled and chopped potatoes

· 1 cup sliced carrots (130 g)

Directions:

Wash the beans and put them along with the other ingredients in the slow cooker.

Nutritional Information: 195 calories, 10 g fat, 13 g amino, 11 g protein

---

7.8 Roasted Beans, Parsnips & Garlic

Time spent on preparation: 5mins

Time spent on cooking: 10mins

Level of Difficulty: Easy

Serving: 2

Ingredients:

· Green beans, eight oz., sliced into 2-inch chunks

· Eight oz. peeled, parsnips

· Eight garlic cloves (only peeled)

· One and a half-cup of extra virgin olive oil

· 1/2 teaspoon tarragon leaves, dried

· A half teaspoon of salt

Directions:

Set the oven temperature to 425 degrees Fahrenheit. Spread the beans, parsnips, and garlic on a foil-lined baking sheet. Pour the oil over the top, flipping gently to cover in a single layer and arrange. 15 minutes of roasting, or until the edges start to brown. Tarragon and salt should be uniformly distributed. Note: If time permits, enclose veggies in foil and set aside 5 minutes to absorb flavors and enable all-natural juices to form.

Nutritional Information: 129 calories, 10 g fat, 13 g amino, 11 g protein

7.9 Cheddar with Black Olives

Time spent on preparation: 10mins

Time spent on cooking: 10mins

Level of Difficulty: Easy

Serving: 2

Ingredients:

· Seven black Greek olives (Greek olives)

· 1 oz. cheddar cheese slice

Directions:

Dice the cheese and insert it into the olive's hole.

Could you put it in your mouth and savor it?

Nutritional Information: 193 calories, 13 g fat, 16 g amino, 24 g protein

---

7.10 Bulgur Almond & Coconut Side

Time spent on preparation: 10mins

Time spent on cooking: 10mins

Level of Difficulty: Easy

Serving: 2

Ingredients:

· 2 oz. almonds, slivered

· 1 quart of water

· 1/3 cup bulgur (dry)

· Two teaspoons of raisin

· Two tablespoons of sweetened flaked coconut

· 1/4 teaspoon cumin powder

· A pinch of cayenne (optional)

· Salt (1/4 teaspoon)

Directions:

Heat the butter over low heat in a medium-sized pot, bringing mild to intense heat. Almonds should be heated for two to three minutes, stirring often, or until golden. Place the pan on a different dish after turning off the heat.

Bring the water, bulgur, and raisins to a boil in a saucepan over high heat. Next, reduce the heat to medium-low, cover, and simmer the mixture for 12 minutes, or until the bulgur is soft. Mix the almonds and the other ingredients in a mixing bowl.

Nutritional Information: 210 calories, 13 g fat, 16 g amino, 24 g protein

7.11 Turnips & Mashed Potatoes

Time spent on preparation: 5mins

Time spent on cooking: 5mins

Level of Difficulty: Easy

Serving: 2

Ingredients:

· 2 lbs. potatoes

· Turnips, peeled and sliced into 1-inch cubes,

· 1 1/2 pounds of chicken broth

· 5 1/4 cups fat-free evaporated milk

· 1/4 cup unsalted butter

· 1/2 tsp. black pepper

Directions:

Mix potatoes, turnips, and broth in a slow cooker. 8-10 hours on low or 6-7 hours on hot. 3 to 4 hours, covered.

Drain part of the cooking liquid and set aside. Using a potato masher, mash the veggies in a bowl. Mix milk and butter in a small pot.

Cook until the butter has melted and the milk is simmering. Stir well after adding the pepper to the potato mixture.

Nutritional Information: 219 calories, 13 g fat, 16 g amino, 24 g protein

---

7.12 Smokey Dipping Potato Fries

Time spent on preparation: 10mins

Time spent on cooking: 10mins

Level of Difficulty: Easy

Serving: 2

Ingredients:

· 1/4 cup plain Greek yogurt (nonfat)

· 1/4 cup mayonnaise (light)

· Ketchup, 1 tbsp.

· Smoked paprika, 1/4 tsp

· A quarter tsp of salt

· Potatoes

· 1 pound peeled sweet potatoes

· 1 tbsp. rapeseed oil

· Salt (1/4 teaspoon)

· One teaspoon of cayenne pepper

Directions:

Set the oven's temperature to 425 degrees. In the meantime, put the sauce's components on a dish and set it away.

On a foil-filled baking sheet, arrange the potatoes in a single layer, drizzle with oil, sprinkle with salt, and bake for 15 minutes or until fork-tender.

Nutritional Information: 160 calories, 10 g fat, 13 g amino, 11 g protein

---

CHAPTER 8

CONDIMENTS AND SAUCES RECIPES

8.1 Indian Mango Chutney

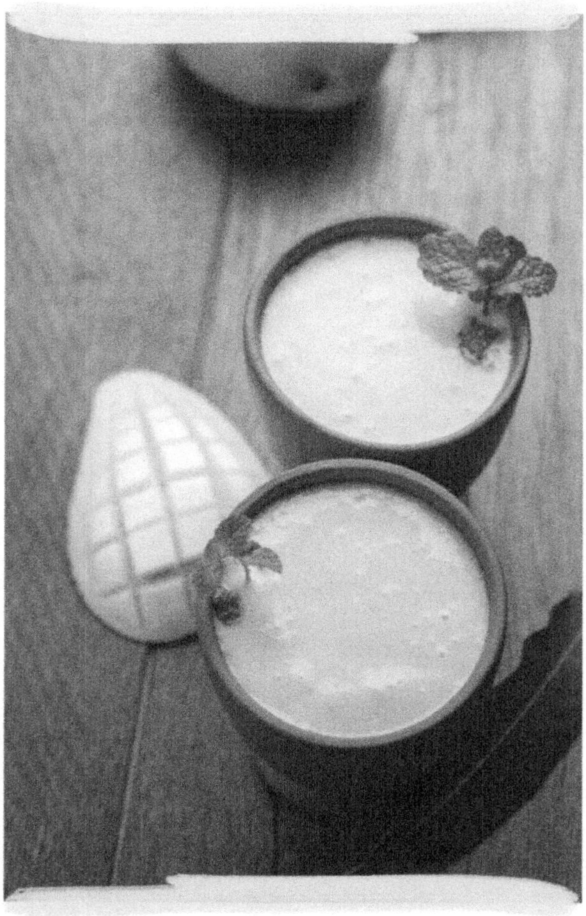

Time spent on preparation: 0 mins

Time spent on cooking: 10 mins

Level of Difficulty: Easy

Serving: 2

Ingredients:

- Three peeled and sliced mangoes (about 2 cups)
- One peeled and chopped tiny yellow onion
- 1/2 cup raisins golden
- One seeded and minced jalapeno pepper
- One tablespoon of rice syrup (brown)
- One lime's zest and two limes' juice
- 2 tbsp. ginger, grated

Directions:

Bring all the ingredients and 12 cups of water to a boil in a large saucepan over high heat.

Reduce the temperature to a moderate setting and cook, uncovered until the sauce has thickened, about 15 minutes.

Nutritional Information: 292 calories, 13 g fat, 16 g amino, 24 g protein

8.2 Strawberry Sauce with Pink Peppermint

Time spent on preparation: 10mins

Time spent on cooking: 10mins

Level of Difficulty: Easy

Serving: 2

Ingredients:

- 2 cups strawberries, chopped

- peppermint hard candies
- 1 cup of water
- A quarter tea pour of peppermint oil

Directions:

In a small mixing bowl, combine the strawberries, candies, water, and extract.

Cover and chill for 1 hour. (Please keep in mind that the mixture may thicken significantly.) Serve over angel food cake, ripe pear pieces, or frozen low-fat vanilla yoghurt.

Nutritional Information: 292 calories, 13 g fat, 16 g amino, 24 g protein

---

8.3 Honey & Mustard Sauce

Time spent on preparation: 10mins

Time spent on cooking: 10mins

Level of Difficulty: Easy

Serving: 2

Ingredients:

- 1/2 cup mustard (prepared)
- 1/4 cup maple pancake syrup (stevia-free)
- tbsp. of mayonnaise
- One tablespoon of Splenda granules

Directions:

Before eating, combine all the ingredients in a mixing dish, cover it, and refrigerate for several hours.

Nutritional Information: 118 calories, 6 g fat, 2 g amino, 4 g protein

---

8.4 Country Veggie Sauce with Chunks

Time spent on preparation: 10mins

Time spent on cooking: 10mins

Level of Difficulty: Easy

Serving: 4

Ingredients:

- 4 ounces sliced mushrooms
- One big red bell pepper, finely chopped
- One moderate yellow squash
- 1 cup chopped onion,
- 1/2 cup frozen carrots,
- Two minced moderate garlic cloves
- 12 coarsely chopped kalamata olives
- 1/3 cup basil leaves, chopped
- 1 tbsp. extra virgin olive oil
- 1 tsp fresh rosemary, chopped
- A half tsp of salt

Directions:

Mix the tomatoes, bell pepper, mushrooms, squash,

onions, carrots, and garlic in a large pot. Stir, cover, and simmer for 30 minutes or until the sauce thickens and the onions soften. Bring to a boil over medium-high heat. Then, reduce to medium-low heat.

Remove from heat, whisk in the other ingredients, and set aside for 5 minutes, coated, to allow flavours to emerge. Serve over baked potatoes, brown rice, or multigrain pasta. If preferred, serve over grilled chicken or fish.

Nutritional Information: 100 calories, 6 g fat, 2 g amino, 4 g protein

---

8.5 Tartar Sauce

Time spent on preparation: 10 mins

Time spent on cooking: 10 mins

Degree of Difficulty: Easy

Serving: 2

Ingredients:

- One tablespoon mayonnaise
- 1 tbsp. sweet pickle relish (stevia-free)
- Lemon juice (two teaspoons)
- Two tablespoons onion, shredded
- One tablespoon mustard (prepared)
- One tablespoon of Splenda granules
- One teaspoon of dill (dried)
- A half teaspoon of Garlic salt with parsley from Lowry
- A quarter teaspoon of black pepper

Directions:

Mix all ingredients, ensuring the Splenda is thoroughly dissolved. Refrigerate for up to four days if kept covered.

Nutritional Information: 120 calories, 6 g fat, 2 g amino, 4 g protein

---

8.6 Red-Pepper Dip

Time spent on preparation: 0 mins

Time spent on cooking: 10 mins

Degree of Difficulty: Easy

Serving: 2

Ingredients:

- 1/2 pound red peppers
- 1/2 cup farmers' cheese
- Extra virgin olive oil or avocado oil, one tablespoon
- 1/2 tablespoon minced garlic
- lemon juice, salt, basil, oregano, and red pepper flakes

Directions:

Peppers should be roasted. Cover and set aside for

15 minutes to cool. Peppers should be seeded and stemmed before peeling them. Prepare the peppers by chopping them.

Garlic and peppers should be combined in a food processor and run until smooth. Garlic and farmers' cheese should be thoroughly blended.

While the machine is running, drizzle in the olive oil and squeeze in the lemon juice; process until smooth before incorporating the basil, oregano, red pepper flakes, and salt. Adjust the spice to taste. After pouring into a basin, refrigerate.

Nutritional Information: 292 calories, 13 g fat, 16 g amino, 24 g protein

---

8.7 Sugar-free Soy Sauce

Time spent on preparation: 10 mins

Time spent on cooking: 10 mins

Serving: 2

Degree of Difficulty: Easy

Ingredients:

- 1 tbsp. soy sauce
- Apple cider vinegar, 2 tbsp.
- 1 tbsp. mustard (stone-ground)
- One teaspoon of ginger, minced
- 1 to 2 garlic cloves, peeled and minced
- 1/2 teaspoon chipotle powder, ground
- 1/2 tsp. paprika (smoked paprika)
- 1/2 teaspoon black pepper, freshly ground
- A quarter teaspoon of onion powder
- Cayenne pepper (1/4 teaspoon)

Directions:

In a blender, place all ingredients and mix on high until creamy.

Nutritional Information: 100 calories, 6 g fat, 2 g amino, 4 g protein

---

8.8 Cauliflower Béchamel

Time spent on preparation: 10 mins

Time spent on cooking: 10 mins

Degree of Difficulty: Easy

Serving: 2

Ingredients:

- One cauliflower head, sliced into florets (approximately 3 cups) (about 3 cups)
- Plain, unsweetened almond milk
- One medium peeled and sliced yellow onion small
- garlic cloves, peeled and minced
- tablespoons thyme, minced

- 1/4 cup basil, finely chopped
- 1/4 teaspoon powdered nutmeg

Directions:

Cauliflower should be placed in a large saucepan partly filled with water.

The cauliflower should be extremely mushy after 10 minutes of simmering after bringing it to a boil over high heat.

In a large frying pan or pot, sauté the onion for 10 minutes at medium heat. To keep the onions from sticking to the pan, add one to two teaspoons of water at a time. Stir in the basil, thyme, and garlic, and cook for one more minute. Cook for five minutes.

In order to get the correct smoothness, if necessary, add up to 12 cups of water to the onion-garlic mixture before blending it with the cauliflower puree.

Nutritional Information: 292 calories, 13 g fat, 16 g amino, 24 g protein

---

8.9 Cranberry Apple Sauce

Time spent on preparation: 10 mins

Time spent on cooking: 10 mins

Degree of Difficulty: Easy

Serving: 2

Ingredients:

- Six peeled or unpeeled apples, diced into 1-inch (2.5 cm) chunks
- 1/2 cup juice from an apple
- 1/2 cup cranberries in season
- 1/4 cup stevia
- A quarter teaspoon of cinnamon

Directions:

In a slow cooker, mix all of the ingredients.

Apples should be cooked over low heat for three to four hours.

Nutritional Information: 292 calories, 13 g fat, 16 g amino, 24 g protein

---

8.10 Chinese Brown Sauce

Time spent on preparation: 10 mins

Time spent on cooking: 10 mins

Degree of Difficulty: Easy

Serving: 2

Ingredients:

- 1/3 cup soy sauce (low sodium)
- 1/4 cup date molasses or brown rice syrup 13 cup vegetable stock or low-sodium vegetable broth
- 1 tbsp. ginger, grated
- garlic cloves, peeled and minced

- Two tablespoons powdered arrowroot

Directions:

All ingredients should be combined in a medium pot and simmered for about 5 minutes over a moderate temperature until hardened. Freeze for up to a week by placing it in an airtight container

Nutritional Information: 172 calories, 15 g fat, 9 g amino, 21 g protein

---

8.11 Horseradish Sauce

Time spent on preparation: 10 mins

Time spent on cooking: 10 mins

Degree of Difficulty: Easy

Serving: 2

Ingredients:

Plain yogurt (8 oz.) (carton)

mayonnaise (1/2 cup)

green onion, 1/4 cup (finely chopped)

One teaspoon of dill weed and two teaspoons of horseradish (dried)

Direction:

Toss the ingredients together in a medium mixing basin. Chill for at least an hour. Serve with thoroughly cooked cold ham.

Nutritional Information: 100 calories, 6 g fat, 2 g amino, 4 g protein

---

8.12 Cocktail Sauce

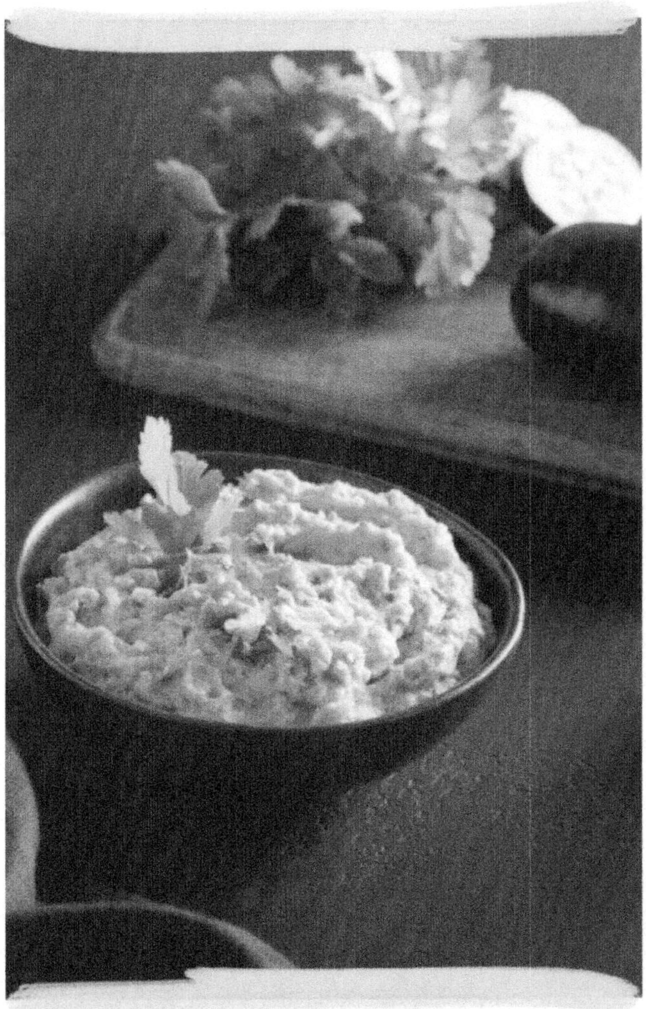

Time spent on preparation: 10 mins

Time spent on cooking: 10 mins

Degree of Difficulty: Easy

Serving: 2

Ingredients:

Ketchup, 1 cup

tablespoons lime juice, three tablespoons grated

horseradish

tablespoons Splenda granulated

1/2 teaspoon spicy sauce from Louisiana

Directions:

Combine all ingredients and keep refrigerated and covered.

Nutritional Information: 130 calories, 6 g fat, 2 g amino, 4 g protein

CHAPTER 9

DESSERTS RECIPES

9.1 Cinnamon Pie Crust

Time spent preparing: 5 minutes

Cook for 60 minutes.

Degree of Difficulty: Easy

Serving: 2

Ingredients:

- 1/4 teaspoon salt
- One teaspoon of Sucralose sweetener
- One teaspoon of cinnamon
- 1/2 cup cold unsalted butter, cubed
- 1/3 cup low-carb all-purpose baking mix
- 4-6 tbsp.sugar-free fruit jam
- 1 beaten egg

Directions:

Combine baking mix, cinnamon, and stevia substitute in a food processor.

Thirty seconds of pulsing. Toss in the butter. Pulse until you get a gritty crumble.

pulse and drip the water gradually until a dough forms. Pulse for another 30 seconds or until everything is well blended.

Wrap the dough in plastic wrap after it has been formed. Wrap into a 3-inch disc and set aside.

Put aside to cool for 30 minutes.

Set the oven's temperature to 400 degrees.

6–8 3 x 3 14-inch thick squares should be cut out of the dough. On a cookie sheet with parchment paper, spread out the dough.

Toss in 1 tablespoon of fruit preserves. Egg wash (egg beaten in a basin) should be used to dap the edges. Place a piece of dough on top of the bottom square. To seal the edges, press down with a fork. Allow the steam to escape by piercing the top of the dough.

Wait 20 minutes before serving until the top is golden brown.

Nutritional Information: 192 calories, 6 g fat, 9 g amino, 20 g protein

---

9.2 Coconut & Lime Mousse

Time spent on preparation: 5 mins

Time spent on cooking: 20 mins

Degree of Difficulty: Easy

Serving: 2

Ingredients:

- Four oz. crème fraiche
- 4 tbsp. stevia extract

- a quarter cup of lime juice
- coconut extract
- 2 quarts cream
- 1/2 cup coconut flakes (unsweetened) for sprinkling

Directions:

With a hand mixer, blend the cream cheese and stevia until well combined before mixing in the lime juice.

Beat in the heavy cream and coconut extract (or vanilla if coconut isn't available) until frothy.

Divide the mixture into four portions; top with unsweetened coconut flakes if preferred.

Nutritional Information: 299 calories, 6 g fat, 9 g amino, 20 g protein

---

9.3 Mango & Pineapple Sorbet

Time spent on preparation: 5 mins

Time spent on cooking: 20 mins

Degree of Difficulty: Easy

Serving: 2

Ingredients:

- Four frozen chopped mango
- 1/2 (8-ounce) can of crushed pineapple, unsweetened
- 1 1/2 tea pours lime juice, freshly squeezed

Directions:

Purée each item in a blender until it is completely smooth

Serve as a sorbet right now, or pour equal quantities into 4 Popsicle moulds and freeze for 4 hours.

Nutritional Information: 290 calories, 6 g fat, 9 g amino, 20 g protein

---

9.4 Pumpkin Pecan Pie Ice cream

Time spent preparing: 5 minutes

Cooking time: 10 minutes

Degree of Difficulty: Easy

Serving: 2

Ingredients:

- 1/2 cup country cheese
- 1/2 cup pureed pumpkin
- 2 quarts coconut cream
- Three big yolks of eggs
- 1/2 teaspoon Xanthan gum
- 20 mL Stevia liquid
- 1 tsp. maple extract (pure)
- One teaspoon of pumpkin pie spice
- 1/2 cup chopped toasted pecans

- 2 tbsp. butter (salted)

Directions:

In a pan, melt some butter. The pecans should be toasted in an oven preheated to 350°F. Before serving, allow cooling.

Combine the cottage cheese, pumpkin puree, coconut cream, and egg yolks separately. To combine the ingredients, whip out the electric mixer.

Combine toasted pecans, xanthan gum, pumpkin spice, liquid stevia, and maple extract in a mixing bowl.

Place the mixture in an ice cream maker and let it stand.

Churn according to the ice cream machine's directions. Serve.

Nutritional Information: 270 calories, 6 g fat, 9 g amino, 20 g protein

---

9.5 Vegan Chocolate Cake

Time spent on preparation: 10 mins

Time spent on cooking: 40 mins

Degree of Difficulty: Easy

Serving: 2

Ingredients:

- 1 cup flour made from spelt
- 1 cup flour made from oats
- 1/2 tbsp. baking soda
- Sucanat (3/4 cups)
- 1/3 cup cocoa powder
- One ripe banana, peeled and mashed
- 1 quart of almond milk
- One teaspoon extract de vanilla
- One teaspoon of vinegar
- egg substitutes
- Silken tofu, 9 oz.
- 12 cups cashews, chopped
- Cocoa powder, two rounded teaspoons
- 14 cup agave nectar
- One teaspoon extract de vanilla

Directions:

The cake needs to be baked at 350 degrees Fahrenheit, so turn on the oven now.

In a large mixing basin, combine the flour, baking soda, cocoa powder, dry sweetener, and cocoa.

In a separate dish, combine the banana, milk, vanilla, vinegar, and egg substitutes.

Make a thorough mix. Mix thoroughly after adding to the flour mixture.

In a 9-inch nonstick baking pan, bake compound for 30 minutes, or until a toothpick inserted in the center comes out clean.

Waiting for the cooking time, make the frosting by processing tofu, cashews, cocoa, agave, and vanilla in a food processor until it is smooth and creamy while the cake cools. Sprinkle evenly over the cake's top.

Nutritional Information: 390 calories, 6 g fat, 9 g amino, 20 g protein

---

9.6 Strawberry Pie

Time spent on preparation: 10 mins

Time spent on cooking: 60 mins

Degree of Difficulty: Moderate

Serving: 2

Ingredients:

- 12 cups fresh strawberries, sliced
- Graham Cracker Crust
- 3/4 cups of water
- 1 cup whole strawberries, frozen (or fresh)
- A quarter cup (organic) cornstarch
- Sucanat, 1/3 cup

Directions:

Fresh, sliced strawberries are layered on top of the graham cracker crust.

Take 1 cup of fresh or frozen strawberries, and simmer them in a medium pot with 3/4 cup water until they are completely dissolved. Mix cornstarch and Sucanat in a mixing bowl and stir into boiling strawberries.

Stir the mixture over medium-low heat, stirring often, for 3–4 minutes, or until it thickens.

Pour the thickened mixture into the pie plate over the cut strawberries.

Nutritional Information: 372 calories, 6 g fat, 9 g amino, 20 g protein

9.7 Chocolate Cherry Ice cream

Time spent on preparation: 10 mins

Time spent on cooking: 1 hour

Degree of Difficulty: Easy

Serving: 2

Ingredients:

- 1/2 cup soy, hemp, or almond milk, vanilla
- 2 tbsp. cocoa powder (natural, non-alkalized)
- dates with pits
- 1/2 cup frozen dark delicious cherries
- One pod of vanilla bean

Directions:

To make the mixture smooth and creamy, combine all the ingredients in a powerful blender or food processor. The vanilla bean should be split lengthwise and rolled open.

With a knife or spoon, scrape the pulp and seeds from within the pod and put them in the blender.

If using a typical blender, blend the first half of the cherries until smooth before adding the remaining cherries and blending once more.

Instead of cherries, you may use frozen berries or a banana. Ripe bananas should be frozen at least 12 hours ahead of time.

Peel bananas split into thirds, and cover them securely in plastic wrap to freeze.

Nutritional Information: 279 calories, 6 g fat, 9 g amino, 20 g protein

---

9.8 Custard Ice cream

Time spent on preparation: 10 mins

Time spent on cooking: 1 hour

Degree of Difficulty: Easy

Serving: 2

Ingredients:

- 3 quarts of thick cream
- 3 beaten egg yolks (large)
- One egg, whole (large)
- 3/4 stevia replacement (sucralose based)
- 1/8 teaspoon of salt
- a half teaspoon of vanilla extract

Directions:

Heat cream in a heavy pot until bubbles appear around the rims. Whisk together the egg, yolks, salt, and stevia substitute while the cream cooks.

Whisk the cream into the eggs slowly and return to the pan. Stirring continuously, cook over medium-low heat for 1 to 2 minutes, or until the mixture thickens enough to cover the back of the spoon.

Take the pan from the heat and dump the contents into a separate basin. Pour in the vanilla extract.

Wrap in plastic and place in the refrigerator for four hours, or until totally cold. While not in use, freeze.

Nutritional Information: 283 calories, 6 g fat, 9 g amino, 20 g protein

---

9.9 Coconut Mango Pudding

Time spent on preparation: 10 mins

Time spent on cooking: 30 mins

Degree of Difficulty: Easy

Serving: 2

Ingredients:

- 1/4 cup quick-cook
- 1/4 teaspoon salt pearl tapioca
- One unsweetened 15-ounce can of coconut milk
- 1 cup sliced mangoes (fresh or frozen)
- Sucanat (12 cups)
- 1/2 gallon soy milk
- One teaspoon extract de vanilla
- A quarter teaspoon of cinnamon

- 14 teaspoon ginger powder

Directions:

In a moderate saucepan, mix the tapioca, salt, coconut milk, mangos, and Sucanat. Bring to a boil, lower to low heat and keep stirring for five minutes.

Mix the soy milk, vanilla, cinnamon, and ginger in a bowl. Return to a boil for three minutes, stirring regularly, then remove from heat.

Nutritional Information: 382 calories, 6 g fat, 9 g amino, 20 g protein

---

9.10 Swedish Apple Pie

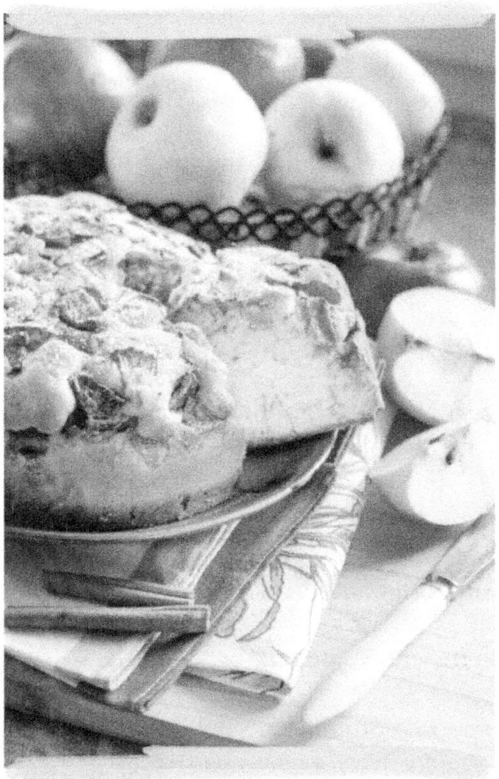

Time spent on preparation: 10 mins

Time spent on cooking: 60 mins

Degree of Difficulty: Moderate

Serving: 2

Ingredients:

- 1/4 cup whole wheat flour 1/2 cup stevia
- 1/4 cup flour (all-purpose)
- One teaspoon of powdered baking soda
- • 1/2 teaspoon salt
- • 1/2 a teaspoon cinnamon powder
- A single huge egg
- A quarter teaspoon of vanilla extract
- chopped medium tart apples
- 3/4 cup toasted chopped walnuts or pecans
- Optional: confectioners' stevia

Directions:

In a large mixing bowl, combine the stevia, flour, baking soda, salt, and cinnamon. Combine the egg and vanilla essence in a separate bowl. Stir the wet ingredients in just enough to moisten the dry ones. Apples and walnuts should be combined in a large mixing dish.

Put the dish in a pie plate with a 9-inch diameter that has been coated with cooking spray. Bake for 25 to 30 minutes, or until a toothpick inserted in the center comes out clean, in a 350°F oven. Dust with confectioners' stevia, if preferred. Before serving, reheat the dish.

Nutritional Information: 302 calories, 6 g fat, 9 g amino, 20 g protein

9.11 Chocolate Pudding

Time spent on preparation: 10 mins

Time spent on cooking: 60 mins

Degree of Difficulty: Moderate

Serving: 2

Ingredients:

- 1 pound of cashews
- 1 quart of water
- A third cup of maple syrup
- One-third of a cup of cocoa powder
- Vanilla extract (two tablespoons)
- Xanthan gum, 1 tbsp.
- 1/2 tsp. mint extract

Directions:

To make everything creamy and smooth, mix all the ingredients in a food processor and pulse several times.

Before serving, chill for at least 2 hours or until thickened.

Nutritional Information: 281 calories, 6 g fat, 9 g amino, 20 g protein

---

9.12 Brownies with chocolate

Time spent on preparation: 10 mins

Time spent on cooking: 30 mins

Degree of Difficulty: Easy

Serving: 2

Ingredients:

- 6 oz. dark chocolate squares
- One stick of butter
- 1 quart of thick cream
- a dozen big eggs
- One stevia cup
- Two tablespoons of powdered baking soda
- Four portions of Atkins flour blend

Directions:

The oven should be preheated to 335 degrees.

Heat the butter and chocolate in a medium microwave-safe dish; alternatively, melt the butter and chocolate on the stovetop and then put in a medium bowl.

Stir the mixture to ensure the chocolate is thoroughly melted.

Heavy cream should be added and combined by whisking.

Whisk together whole eggs and stevia substitute in a mixing basin until combined.

Put it into the chocolate mixture at moderate speed.

Using a spoon, combine the Atkins flour mix and baking powder.

Using cooking spray, coat a medium baking pan.

Ensure that the batter is spread equally throughout the pan.

Bake in the oven at 350 degrees for 30 to 35 minutes.

After removing the brownies from the oven, let them cool on a cooling rack.

After it is safe to handle, cut it into pieces.

Place the cookies on a tray or in an airtight container.

Put the food on the table.

Nutritional Information: 382 calories, 6 g fat, 9 g amino, 20 g protein

CHAPTER 10

DRINKS RECIPES

10.1 Basic Fruit Smoothie

Time spent on preparation: 10 mins

Time spent on cooking: 10 mins

Degree of Difficulty: Easy

Serving: 2

Ingredients:

- One can of navy beans
- 12 quarts of orange juice
- 2 cups fresh or frozen strawberries or blueberries, quartered
- Two teaspoons of granulated stevia sweetener
- 1/2 tablespoons cinnamon powder
- 1/8 teaspoon nutmeg

powder

- 6–8 ice cubes, as required (optional)

Directions:

In a mixer, puree all ingredients (excluding the ice cubes) until smooth. If using fresh fruits, mix with ice until completely smooth.

Nutritional Information: 178 calories, 13 g fat, 16 g amino, 24 g protein

---

10.2 Basic Vegetable Juice

Time spent on preparation: 0 mins

Time spent on cooking: 5 mins

Degree of Difficulty: Easy

Serving: 2

Ingredients:

- 3/4 cup walnuts, chopped
- 1/2 cup tomatoes, crumbled
- Two tablespoons salsa (mild or spicy)
- One seeded dribbled and quartered red bell pepper
- 1 tbsp. finely chopped zucchini
- One green onion, finely cut
- One celery stalk, chopped
- 1/2 tiny chopped jalapeno chillies
- One teaspoon of granulated stevia sweetener
- One teaspoon of black pepper, freshly ground
- 1/8 teaspoon cloves, ground

Directions:

Batch-process all contents in a stick blender on high until finely chopped. If required, add a little water slowly to get the right consistency.

Nutritional Information: 172 calories, 15 g fat, 9 g amino, 21 g protein

---

10.3 Tropical Tea

Time spent on preparation: 0 mins

Time spent on cooking: 5 mins

Degree of Difficulty: Easy

Serving: 2

Ingredients:

- 6 quarts (1.4 litres) of boiling water
- Tea bags (six)
- 1/3 cup stevia (67 g)
- tablespoons honey (40 g)
- Orange juice, 112 cups (355 ml)
- Pineapple juice, 112 cups (355 ml)
- One sliced orange

Directions:

Fill the tea bags halfway with boiling water.

Five minutes are required after covering. Mix the remaining ingredients. Heat on low for 2 to 3 hours in a slow cooker.

Nutritional Information: 292 calories, 13 g fat, 16 g amino, 24 g protein

---

10.4 Spiced Tea

Time spent on preparation: 0 mins

Time spent on cooking: 5 mins

Degree of Difficulty: Easy

Serving: 2

Ingredients:

- 1 cup instant tea (32 g)
- cups quick orange drink mix (416 g)
- 1 cup stevia (200 g)
- tablespoons lemonade mix (28 g)
- 1 tbsp. ground cloves (6.6 g)
- 1 tbsp. (7 g) cinnamon powder

Directions:

Mix all ingredients in an airtight jar and store. In a slow cooker, pour 14 cups (50 g) of the mix for each quart (960 ml) of water.

Heat on low until the mixture is warm, stirring regularly to ensure the powder is completely dissolved.

Nutritional Information: 147 calories, 13 g fat, 16 g amino, 24 g protein

---

10.5 Smoothie with pumpkin pie

Time spent on preparation: 10 mins

Time spent on cooking: 10 mins

Serving: 2

Degree of Difficulty: Easy

Ingredients:

- 1 cup almond milk (unsweetened) or water
- 1/2 cup pureed pumpkin
- Ice cubes (12 cups)
- • A quarter-teaspoon of pure vanilla essence 4 pitted and sliced Medjool dates, or more to your liking
- 1/4 teaspoon cinnamon powder
- 1 tsp. nutmeg, ground

Directions:

Purée all of the ingredients in a mixer until they are creamy and smooth.

Nutritional Information: 158 calories, 13 g fat, 16 g amino, 24 g protein

---

10.6 Mexican Hot Chocolate

Time spent on preparation: 10 mins

Time spent on cooking: 10 mins

Degree of Difficulty: Easy

Serving: 2

Ingredients:

- 1/4 cup chocolate powder, unsweetened
- 1/4 cup stevia sweetener or agave syrup
- 3/4 teaspoon cinnamon powder
- A quarter teaspoon of salt
- 4 cups soy milk

Directions:

In a small dish, combine the salt, 3/4 tsp. cinnamon, stevia or syrup, cocoa, and chocolate powder. In a saucepan, heat one cup of milk until bubbles start to appear around the pan's edges.

Once the cocoa mixture has been added, whisk it in well. Bring to a simmer while stirring often over a low burner.

Ring to a simmer with the remaining 3 cups of milk. Take the pan from the heat and quickly pour it into serving glasses. Dust with cinnamon and a dollop of whipped topping on top of each.

Nutritional Information: 293 calories, 13 g fat, 16 g amino, 24 g protein

---

10.7 Kale Smoothie

Time spent on preparation: 10 mins

Time spent on cooking: 10 mins

Degree of Difficulty: Easy

Serving: 2

Ingredients:

- 1 cup cleaned and chopped fresh kale or baby spinach
- 1 pound of strawberries (
- 1/2 avocado
- 1/2 lemon or lime juice
- 2–3 kiwifruit, peeled

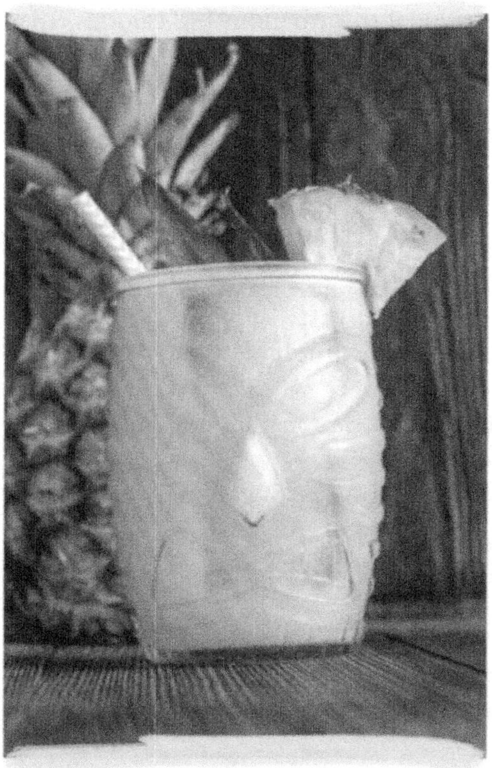

Directions:

Blend all the ingredients together in a blender until they are completely smooth.

Pour into mugs and top with a strawberry slice if desired.

Nutritional Information: 177 calories, 13 g fat, 16 g amino, 24 g protein

---

10.8 Fruit & Tofu Smoothie

Time spent on preparation: 0 mins

Time spent on cooking: 5 mins

Degree of Difficulty: Easy

Serving: 2

Ingredients:

- 1 cup tofu (silky soft tofu)
- One peeled banana halved crosswise
- 1/2 cup orange juice or soy milk
- 1/2 cup vanilla low-fat yoghurt
- 1/4 cup strawberries or blueberries, fresh or frozen
- a quarter cup of wheat germ
- One tablespoon of granulated stevia sweetener

Directions:

Mix the tofu, one banana half, soy milk or orange juice, and yoghurt until smooth.

Mix in the berries and wheat germ one more. Blend in the remaining banana half and the stevia until smooth. Serve right away.

Nutritional Information: 256 calories, 13 g fat, 16 g amino, 24 g protein

---

10.9 Pina Colada

Time spent on preparation: 0 mins

Time spent on cooking: 5 mins

Degree of Difficulty: Easy

Serving: 2

Ingredients:

- 1 1/2 pounds of ice
- pineapple juice or 1/2 cup chopped pineapple (frozen)
- Coconut cream by Coco Lopez
- White and black rum, 1.5 oz.

Directions:

Blend the ice, coconut cream, frozen pineapple, juice, and both white and black rums in a blender. Mix the ingredients until they are frosty and smooth.

Place pineapple slices on the rims of two glasses after pouring the drink into them.

Nutritional Information: 272 calories, 13 g fat, 16 g amino, 24 g protein

10.10 Peach Apricot Sorbet

Time spent on preparation: 0 mins

Time spent on cooking: 5 mins

Degree of Difficulty: Easy

Serving: 2

Ingredients:

- 2 cups peaches, frozen
- 1/4 cup water or soy, hemp, or almond milk
- dried apricots, chopped, unsweetened and unsulfured

Directions:

In a high-powered blender, combine all ingredients.

Nutritional Information: 142 calories, 13 g fat, 16 g amino, 24 g protein

10.11 Pumpkin Punch

Time spent on preparation: 0 mins

Time spent on cooking: 5 mins

Degree of Difficulty: Easy

Serving: 2

Ingredients:

- 1/2 cup pureed pumpkin
- 1 tsp. spice blend (or cinnamon)
- a half teaspoon of vanilla extract
- 3/4 cup almond milk, unsweetened
- One banana or berries, chilled
- Honey to taste 6-7 ice cubes

Directions:

Blend until smooth in a blender. If preferred,

garnish with mint and nutmeg.

Nutritional Information: 122 calories, 13 g fat, 12 g amino, 6g protein

---

10.12 Banana Matcha Smoothie

Time spent on preparation: 10 mins

Time spent on cooking: 10 mins

Degree of Difficulty: Easy

Serving: 2

Ingredients:

- Cup of fat-free milk (optional)
- 1/4 cup frozen chopped pineapple
- Ice cubes (1/2 cup)
- One tablespoon of powdered Matcha
- 1/4 teaspoon cinnamon powder

Directions:

Combine all of the ingredients in a blender.

To chop the ingredients, pulse the mixture numerous times.

Blend for 30 to 60 seconds or until completely smooth and blended. If desired, sweeten with liquid stevia extract to taste.

Nutritional Information: 142 calories, 13 g fat, 12 g amino, 6g protein

10.13 Vanilla Mixed Berry Smoothie

Time spent on preparation: 10 mins

Time spent on cooking: 10 mins

Degree of Difficulty: Easy

Serving: 2

Ingredients:

- 1/2 cup plain nonfat Greek yoghurt
- 1/2 cup blueberries, frozen
- 1/4 cup strawberries, frozen
- 3–4 ice cubes one teaspoon freshly squeezed lemon juice

Direction:

Combine all the ingredients in a blender.

To chop the ingredients, pulse the mixture numerous times.

Blend for 30 to 60 seconds or until completely smooth and blended.

If desired, sweeten with liquid stevia extract to taste.

Immediately pour into a glass and serve.

Nutritional Information: 164 calories, 13 g fat, 12 g amino, 6g protein

---

10.14 Green Tea Cider Refresher

Time spent on preparation: 10 mins

Time spent on cooking: 10 mins

Degree of Difficulty: Easy

Serving: 2

Ingredients:

- Two teaspoons extra virgin olive oil
- Eight tea bags (green)
- 1 cup heated water
- 2 quarts of cold water
- One tablespoon of apple cider vinegar (no stevia added)
- 1 cup granulated stevia sweetener

Directions:

Tea bags are added after halfway through a 4-quart pitcher of boiling water. To steep, cover and set aside for five minutes.

Mix in the cold water, vinegar, and stevia until the stevia is completely dissolved. Serve with ice cubes.

Nutritional Information: 111 calories, 13 g fat, 12 g amino, 6g protein

---

10.15 Strawberry Chia Seed Milkshake

Time spent on preparation: 10 mins

Time spent on cooking: 10 mins

Degree of Difficulty: Easy

Serving: 2

Ingredients:

- 2 cups of unsweetened coconut or almond milk
- 1/2 cup strawberries, raspberries, and/or blueberries
- chai tea bags, three tablespoons chia seeds, ground
- One tablespoon of honey or maple syrup
- One teaspoon extract de vanilla

Directions:

Discard the tea bags' spices after removing them.

Combine the almond milk, blueberries, chia seeds, honey, vanilla essence, and spices from the chai tea bags and mix until smooth.

Serve chilled.

Nutritional Information: 292 calories, 13 g fat, 16 g amino, 24 g protein

---

30 Day meal plan

WEEK 1

DAY 1:

Breakfast: Banana waffles

Lunch: Tuna fish salad

Dinner: Ground turkey breast and cheese-stuffed tomatoes

Snack: Cheese strips

DAY 2:

Breakfast: Keto cinnamon coffee

Lunch: Keto Cobb salad

Dinner: Classic pork tenderloin

Snack: Homemade butter power granola

DAY 3:

Breakfast: Omelet Caprese

Lunch: 5-ingredient keto salad

Dinner: Succulent chicken parmesan

Snack: Homemade graham breakers

DAY 4:

Breakfast: Banana waffles

Lunch: Tuna fish salad

Dinner: Ground turkey breast and cheese-stuffed tomatoes

Snack: Cheese strips

DAY 5:

Breakfast: Keto cinnamon coffee

Lunch: Keto Cobb salad

Dinner: Classic pork tenderloin

Snack: Homemade butter power granola

DAY 6:

Breakfast: Omelet Caprese

Lunch: 5-ingredient keto salad

Dinner: Succulent chicken parmesan

Snack: Homemade graham breakers

DAY 7:

Breakfast: Banana waffles

Lunch: Tuna fish salad

Dinner: Ground turkey breast and cheese-stuffed tomatoes

Snack: Cheese strips

WEEK 2

DAY 8:

Breakfast: Scrambled fresh eggs

Lunch: Vegetarian keto Cobb

Dinner: Flavorful chicken & mushrooms

Snack: Mozzarella Cheese Pockets

DAY 9:

Breakfast: Omelet of keto cheese

Lunch: Tuna and mushrooms casserole

Dinner: Heartwarming chilli chicken

Snack: No Bake Coconut Cookies

DAY 10:

Breakfast: Keto fresh eggs with ripe avocado and bacon

Lunch: Hearty chicken salad

Dinner: Lamb chops with kale

Snack: Cheesy Cauliflower Breadsticks

DAY 11:

Breakfast: Scrambled fresh eggs

Lunch: Vegetarian keto Cobb

Dinner: Flavorful chicken & mushrooms

Snack: Mozzarella Cheese Pockets

DAY 12:

Breakfast: Omelet of keto cheese

Lunch: Tuna and mushrooms casserole

Dinner: Heartwarming chilli chicken

Snack: No Bake Coconut Cookies

DAY 13:

Breakfast: Keto fresh eggs with ripe avocado and bacon

Lunch: Hearty chicken salad

Dinner: Lamb chops with kale

Snack: Cheesy Cauliflower Breadsticks

DAY 14:

Breakfast: Scrambled fresh eggs

Lunch: Vegetarian keto Cobb

Dinner: Flavorful chicken & mushrooms

Snack: Mozzarella Cheese Pockets

WEEK 3

DAY 15:

Breakfast: Yellow bell pepper, mozzarella, and fresh bacon frittata

Lunch: Mouth-watering Greek salad

Dinner: Scrumptious tartar salmon

Snack: Keto No-Bake Cookies

DAY 16:

Breakfast: Savory cheese sausage pies

Lunch: Zucchini salad

Dinner: Tuna and mushrooms casserole

Snack: Swiss Cheese Crunchy Nachos

DAY 17:

Breakfast: Delicious breakfast tart

Lunch: Arugula and fresh raspberry salad

Dinner: Signature Italian pork dish

Snack: Homemade Thin Mints

DAY: 18

Breakfast: Yellow bell pepper, mozzarella, and fresh bacon frittata

Lunch: Mouth-watering Greek salad

Dinner: Scrumptious tartar salmon

Snack: Keto No-Bake Cookies

DAY 19:

Breakfast: Savory cheese sausage pies

Lunch: Zucchini salad

Dinner: Tuna and mushrooms casserole

Snack: Swiss Cheese Crunchy Nachos

DAY 20:

Breakfast: Delicious breakfast tart

Lunch: Arugula and fresh raspberry salad

Dinner: Signature Italian pork dish

Snack: Homemade Thin Mints

DAY 21:

Breakfast: Yellow bell pepper, mozzarella, and fresh bacon frittata

Lunch: Mouth-watering Greek salad

Dinner: Scrumptious tartar salmon

Snack: Keto No-Bake Cookies

WEEK 4

DAY 22:

Breakfast: Fresh raspberry and cocoa breakfast

Lunch: Romaine lettuce with blueberry mixture

Dinner: Flawless grilled steak

Snack: Easy Peanut Fresh Butter Cups

DAY 23:

Breakfast: Steak & fresh eggs

Lunch: Caesar salad

Dinner: Spiced pork tenderloin

Snack: Cheese Strips

DAY 24:

Breakfast: Scrambled fresh eggs, ricotta cheese

Lunch: Quick tilapia

Dinner: Sticky pork ribs

Snack: Peanut Butter Power Granola

DAY 25:

Breakfast: Fresh raspberry and cocoa breakfast

Lunch: Romaine lettuce with blueberry mixture

Dinner: Flawless grilled steak

Snack: Easy Peanut Fresh Butter Cups

DAY 26:

Breakfast: Steak & fresh eggs

Lunch: Caesar salad

Dinner: Spiced pork tenderloin

Snack: Cheese Strips

DAY 27:

Breakfast: Scrambled fresh eggs, ricotta cheese

Lunch: Quick tilapia

Dinner: Sticky pork ribs

Snack: Peanut Butter Power Granola

DAY 28:

Breakfast: Fresh raspberry and cocoa breakfast

Lunch: Romaine lettuce with blueberry mixture

Dinner: Flawless grilled steak

Snack: Easy Peanut Fresh Butter Cups

WEEK 5

DAY 29:

Breakfast: Chicken omelette California style

Lunch: Quick and easy tuna fish salad

Dinner: Valentine's DAY dinner

Snack: Homemade graham Breakers

DAY 30:

Breakfast: Quick and easy juicer or blender pancakes

Lunch: Taste the chicken salad

Dinner: South East Asian steak platter

Snack: Keto No-Bake Cookies

CONCLUSIONS

he Low-FODMAP diet is an effective method for treating digestive diseases, such as inflammatory bowel disease and irritable bowel syndrome. The diet involves limiting or avoiding high-FODMAP foods, which are carbohydrates that can be difficult to digest for some individuals.

The Low-FODMAP diet can help reduce symptoms such as bloating, gas, abdominal pain, and diarrhea or constipation by identifying and eliminating trigger foods. However, working with a healthcare professional or registered dietitian is important to ensure that the diet is nutritionally balanced and sustainable over the long term.

The Low-FODMAP diet can provide a personalized approach to managing digestive symptoms and offer benefits such as improved quality of life and bowel habits. While it may require some adjustments to eating habits, the diet's potential benefits may be worth it for individuals who struggle with digestive symptoms.